"Magnificent! Whispers in Sound is a triumph!!!

Reading Laura Penn Gallerstein's book is a victory for all! She writes for the householder, the ordinary and the magical. Laura embraces her journey into a life as a beautiful woman in which we all have so much in common. She reminds us how the divine is always with us by opening your intuition, speaking in your dreams and offering you the medicine through sound and light.

Thank you, Laura for giving us the opportunity to take a deep peek into your sacred path. As a reader, I appreciated your thoughtful gifts of awakening for continual enlightenment and healing through your personalized meditations in sound that align with each chapter and for everyday life. Your book is a precious treasure."

– **Mahanraj Kaur "Marcia"**, Owner of Great Divine Flow Yoga

---

"Fantastic book! A healing experience from page i.

Whispers in Sound captures the beauty and power of vibrational medicine. Laura has written an easy to follow manual of inspiration and meditation. I found myself falling in love with my own sound again! Thank you, Laura for being you, walking your path, speaking about it, and giving people an amazing tool for self-empowerment. Your positivity continually lifts us up!"

– **Amanda Dominitz**, Director Soul of Yoga Sound Institute, Owner of Sacred Sound of the Soul

---

"You are in for a page turning memorable and informative read. Enjoy!!!"

Laura has written such a compelling book about her journey to healing, weaving all her discoveries and sharing each turn and twist in her life as she worked carefully to achieve the balance of her mind, body, soul and spirit.

Her honest and authentic personal narrative is a heartwarming, humble and sometimes humorous when she takes us on her many life challenging experiences. Laura will captivate you with her concrete explanations of the power of dreams, guided meditations and the importance of sound in healing!"

– **Pam Laidlaw Ph.D., RN, BN, MA**
In Marriage, Family Therapy, and Ph D in Psychology

"*Whispers in Sound* **is a breakthrough book integrating the challenges of life as a memoir and interweaves healing within each chapter through her lovely meditations.** The author's search for life's meaning and her desire to share her discoveries, both inner and outer, beckons the reader to examine their own life and opens the door to opportunity as they experience a range of effortless meditation practices that ultimately lead to Source."

– **Michele Hébert, E-RYT 500,**
Author *The Tenth Door: A Yoga Adventure*

"**The time is now!** Laura invites us to raise our frequency as we connect to unconditional love individually and together as one on this planet.

Laura shares a journey of remembering, which reveals how life is about discovery in order to authentically understand why we are here on the planet at this time. There are many souls beginning to wake up. Her lifelong search for truth offers a fascinating story of how we must trust the process of our soul's journey and be willing to do the work needed to peel away the layers of false perceptions until we connect to our own sacred presence. Only then can we step up and share our gifts with the world in peace as she describes so eloquently in the book. Thank you, Laura, for doing the work and never giving up!"

– **Flossie Park, E-RYT 500, YACEP,** Sound Healer, Director of 200 Hatha & Gentle Yoga Teacher Trainings, Soul of Yoga, Encinitas, CA

"When I first heard Laura play her beautiful bowls, I immediately felt the vibration right into my heart chakra. I am so grateful for her commitment to write this book. She really is able to exemplify the positive energy of yin, which she lives within, in everything she does. This book is a beautiful expression of her soul.

The soft "whispers" of sound healing help us remember who we were as we connect with the ancient wisdom of our ancestors. I feel vibration and sound healing do open the portal to integrate mind, body and spirit. I will be using these beautiful meditations with my clients, especially with those who have experienced trauma and grief."

– Mary Ellen Capps M.Ed., LPC

"Let this book whisper to you, learn how to hear the sounds, feel the vibrations and tune into your true self. Read *Whispers in Sound* to uncover Laura's spiritual life discoveries that will take you on a reflective journey of introspection. This book will shift your thoughts about the positive impact sound and vibration can have on your life."

– Jill Nussinow, The Veggie Queen™

"Laura's book Whispers in Sound does more than narrate her life story; it shows how we can open to Source, or Spirit as she calls it. Her life is shown as a series of awakenings which help her trust, heal, and ultimately find clarity and wisdom. I love Laura's crystal meditations! They are tenderly written and immediately palpable."

– Wah!, Author of *Self-Care: Building a Smarter, Stronger, More Peaceful Self*

Whispers in Sound

A Profound Healing Journey through Sacred Vibrations and Meditation

Laura Penn Gallerstein

Whispers in Sound
A Profound Healing Journey through Sacred Vibrations and Meditation

Published by:
Sedona Sacred Sounds Press
Sedona, AZ
www.SedonaSacredSoundsPress.com

First Paperback Edition 2021

ISBN's:
978-1-7365593-0-7 (Soft cover)
978-1-7365593-1-4 (Hard cover)
978-1-7365593-2-1 (Mobi Ebook)
978-1-7365593-3-8 (Epub Ebook)

Library of Congress Control Number:
2021910606

Editor: Arlene Matthews
Copy Editor: Jeff Braucher
Cover & Interior Design: Diane Rigoli
Photos: Janise Witt

TABLE OF CONTENTS

FOREWORD

Whispers in Sound is a masterful weave of the author's life experiences—with their ups and downs, highs and lows—intermingled with her search for a meaningful career path. It has been a path that ultimately evolved side by side with, and through, her many challenges.

Body, mind, spirit, and emotion in unison flow through the writer's words, illuminating her choices and practices. Her innate joy and search across many body and mind disciplines took her deeper into spirit and inner understanding of self. Pilates and yoga were deepened by meditations, until she was finally inspired by finding her beloved crystal bowls, which offered her more nuanced healing through sound vibration. Laura personifies, through her searching for meaning in life, Rumi's timeless quote: "That which you are seeking is seeking you."

Whispers in Sound is a beautiful example of how life responds by opening doorways when one goes down its path with an open mind and heart. The author's stories bring authenticity to the practices she describes, relating intrinsically to her emotions in each chapter of her life.... a journey that is still evolving! And the book's sound healing offerings provide very practical and inspiring tools to guide readers on their own journeys.

This book is ultimately a path to living LIFE to the full in the present moment, experientially. It is also a great workbook that points a way to understanding the meaning of Socrates' immortal saying, "The unexamined life is not worth living." Laura illustrates a way to examine your way...offering insight for each reader to weave the challenges of their own life into their own chosen practices, and to live beautifully and fully as a result.

I am so delighted Laura has written this book. It is a shining light on who she is: one of the most joyful people I have ever known (and someone whose laughter always elevates my soul). Humor and love have always been special gift she gives to the world, and they are now joined by this inspiring book based on a life that epitomizes the author's favorite word: Amazing!

– Phyllis Pilgrim
Past Director of Healing The Spirit Program at Rancho La Puerta

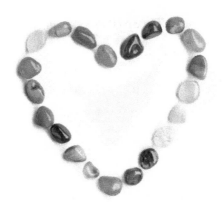

Gary, my husband and best friend, who continues to support me in every way on our journey through life together. From the bottom of my heart, thank you for being my biggest advocate and rock for 30 years and counting!

My Mothers: Etta and Janet
My Father: Mitchell
My Kids: Mitch, Laura and Eric
My Greatest Teachers...

With love I dedicate this book to all of you.

The moment you start acting like life is a blessing,
it starts feeling like one.

– UNKNOWN

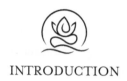

INTRODUCTION

The New GPS

*In the end, only three things matter: how much you loved,
how gently you lived, and how gracefully you
let go of things not meant for you.*

– GAUTAMA BUDDHA

Many years ago my mother, who passed away when I was a girl, came to me in a vivid dream and told me, "It is a blessing to be alive." After that dream, a depression I'd been experiencing subsided, and I started to find my true passion and niche in this world. Now, though, I see there was even more to her message. We—all of us—are so blessed to be alive and to be right here right now, because we are witnesses to the Shift of Ages.

As I write this, we are living through a world crisis, and countless people are experiencing inner crises. This episode is forcing people to examine what is really important, to reconfigure their priorities, and to consider what creates value for them. Making money, although certainly necessary for survival, does not, in itself, create value. We create value by finding our joyful purpose in this life and by using our God-given talents to create from our hearts.

The Dalai Lama, when asked what surprised him most about humanity, answered: "Man. Because he sacrifices his health in order to make money. Then he sacrifices money to recuperate his health. And then he is so anxious about the future that he does not enjoy the present; the result being that he does not live in the present or the future; he lives as if he is never going to die, and then dies having never really lived."

That was true of nearly all of us. But that was before.

Then The Virus hit the planet. The world stopped. And despite all the initial fear and confusion—always by-products of dramatic change—the Age of Aquarius began to dawn more fully. Predicted for years as the coming era of humankind's evolution into a state of higher consciousness on this planet, this so-called Age of Light coincides with a shift from linear thinking to multidimensional thinking, from the constrained analytical mind to the intuitive mind. The analytical mind is good for following orders, but the orders in this new day must come from our hearts and our deeper awareness of Being.

As we cocooned at home, many of us came to the same realization: Going within is what we are being called to do right now on this planet. We are not meant to waste any more time on so many external distractions. As Dr. Mitchell Gaynor said, "It's time to realize who we are and why we are on Earth at this particular transformative time and then share it."

From that point forward, we began being guided by an age-old internal navigation system, which I call the New GPS. This intuitive guidance system is pointing us toward internal rather than external validation. We need to experience this interior validation in order to understand that we are amazing human beings who chose to be born at a time that will catapult our evolution into a higher realm.

We are in for the ride of a lifetime—one that will awaken us to our nearly unlimited potential.

January 2020 began a new year and a new decade—a decade for purging, for clarity, and for truth surfacing everywhere. I could palpably feel the energy, quite different from that of 2019, and I caught glimpses of happenings in the news that told me it was going to be a life-altering year. I could feel the veil between heaven and earth becoming razor thin. I could almost hear the whispers in my ears from my angels. Yet I didn't see yet how it could happen or what I could contribute.

On a personal level I felt I had done a lot of internal work. I had healed so much from the loss of my mom, created loving relationships with my husband, children, and had dissolved a business partnership. I felt ready to soar in a new direction. I consulted with an astrologer I trusted deeply who had insisted there was a book inside me that needed to be published. I had been writing a metaphysical book for children, but I didn't know if that was the one. But I knew that if I remained centered and quiet, messages—which I think of as "downloads"—from my inner guiding voice, which I call Spirit, would come, and I would know just how to proceed.

I had learned throughout the years that when I let go of something, the answer would always come back to me, albeit from an altered perspective or in a different way than I thought it should. In early 2020 I was trusting Spirit more and more than I ever had in my life. I trusted that when things were smooth and flowing, that was an indication that this was the direction to take. I had learned, for the most part, to stop arguing with Spirit and follow the energy of the moment. When I do follow the energy, life feels like a flowing river. When the energy is blocked, I can usually feel the blockage in my gut, tight and uncomfortable. I had also learned that when I pay attention to my dreams, an answer usually follows.

Before long my path became clear to me. In February 2020 I went to Rancho La Puerta, a legendary 80-year-old world-class wellness resort in Baja California, to lead sound healing classes. Over the past ten years I have incorporated guided meditations with alchemy crystal bowls. These bowls bring in healing vibrations because they are attuned to our energy centers and bring recalibration and balance.

My husband Gary and I had a fantastic week, with healing on so many levels for me personally and for many people that came to my classes. We connected with so many amazing, beautiful people who were so encouraging and supportive in such a generous way. I felt as though I were turning into a butterfly, whereas a few months before I'd felt tight in my skin, like a caterpillar. While at the Ranch, as it's referred to, I received quite a few "downloads." I heard, "Write a book with some of your guided meditations from over the years and include a link to soundtrack files so people can hear you play the bowls." While there I started writing this book, and kept writing when I got home.

Back in Sedona, Arizona, I got a clear message to finish the book while life, as we knew it, stopped. It was time to get it done, to publish it, and to send it out into the world. This was it. It felt so urgent, just as the astrologer had said. Every day I sat down and wrote for hours. I also cooked, did yoga, meditated, went hiking, and cleaned house.

One day when I was making the bed as I had done a thousand times before, I looked down into the gap between the box spring and bed frame and saw some dust along the ledge. I asked Gary to get the vacuum hose, and as soon as I turned the vacuum on, something got stuck. To my utter surprise it was my dad's ring, which I thought I had lost months before. Tears of happiness stung my eyes. My heart was so full. I felt that my dad, or my angels, had put the ring there, because there was no way I'd dropped it or felt it drop. I took it as a sign from the spirit world that I was on the right path. My father loved words and writing and had even won a poetry-reading contest when he was young. I was overjoyed that my dad was choosing to help me in such a beautiful, supportive way.

The portents continued. One day while hiking I heard the voice I call Spirit loud and clear: "Where were you when the world stopped?" I said "What?" I heard the question again. And again, and again. I probably heard that query at least five times on my daily hikes. I realized at last that my unseen "team" had pushed the idea of my writing a book when the world stopped. I grew so used to them talking with me that eventually I just said, "I got it loud and clear and thank you." After that, they stopped repeating the phrase. I can't help loving them for all their insistent care and reinforcement. Their persistence, even when I initially resist, reminds me that we are never alone and that we have boundless help available for moving our lives forward in the most positive direction. That help is called Love. Our helpers never stop loving us, knowing we need all the guidance we can possibly get as we walk this earthly journey. Thank goodness we are not alone!

With so many seen and unseen helpers, I was able to complete my writing in less time than I'd thought possible. And now, with gratitude, I am able to offer this book of healing meditations.

These practices represent a culmination of years of receiving messages in dreams, of learning healing tools, of teaching, and of guiding clients into deep states of relaxation. Each meditation is designed for a specific purpose, such as healing relationships, cultivating optimism and inspiration, and increasing self-appreciation and love.

This book can be a resource for you during this special time and, going forward, during any time of change. You can trust your own inner voice to help you pick it up when it is most needed and to choose particular meditations for daily use. Included with this book is a link to soundtracks on which I play alchemy singing bowls to accompany the guided healing meditations. The combination of visualization, guided meditation, and playing the bowls is pure magic. So these soundtracks, too, can become daily companions on your journey of evolving and accessing the multidimensional being that you are.

But this book incorporates other aspects as well. The meditations themselves are preceded by the story of my personal spiritual journey, including life experiences as well as nighttime dreams that have taught and inspired me. I confess that I was not inclined, at first, to augment the meditations in this way. But as the month of March 2020 passed and I became increasingly motivated to continue writing down the meditations, I was surprised when I heard another "download" voice instructing me: "Now tell your personal story along with the meditations."

Silly me, I started arguing with the voice I call Spirit, saying, "No, I really don't want to go down that path."

Spirit said, "You need to do this not only for yourself to heal but for many others to heal."

I argued again. "It's too much work and far too difficult to go back and unravel this story."

Spirit insisted. "You need to do this and now is the time. There is not going to be any other time like this on your planet. This is the time and the opportunity is here now."

Okay, I got it. You can argue with Spirit for just so long. Ultimately I acknowledged that such internal wisdom is always right, and when I stopped digging in my heels, I realized that the instruction made complete sense. And so it was done. My story helped me to move forward on my personal journey; now, I offer it to you to help you awaken to your unseen world of guidance and healing.

In this time of uncertainty, we need many tools for navigating our lives. The world will never be the same. We cannot go back to being self-centered without regard for others. We cannot go back to having work that only supports our financial state. We must understand our own unique purpose. For however many years each of us is destined to live on this beautiful blue-green planet—whether it's twenty, thirty, fifty, or one hundred years—we are meant to use that time wisely. We can only go forward on our path. There is no return to what was. We truly are in for a magical voyage.

Enjoy these meditations, and hopefully they will help you work out whatever needs to be worked out for your highest healing and growth. How will you know if they are working? Give them some time, and you may see that your life becomes filled with synchronous moments daily and that small miracles begin to happen. This is not due to me, of course, nor to any external force. Rather, it all emanates from tapping into your creativity. That is the doorway to your heart and to the quiet voice inside of you—to the New GPS.

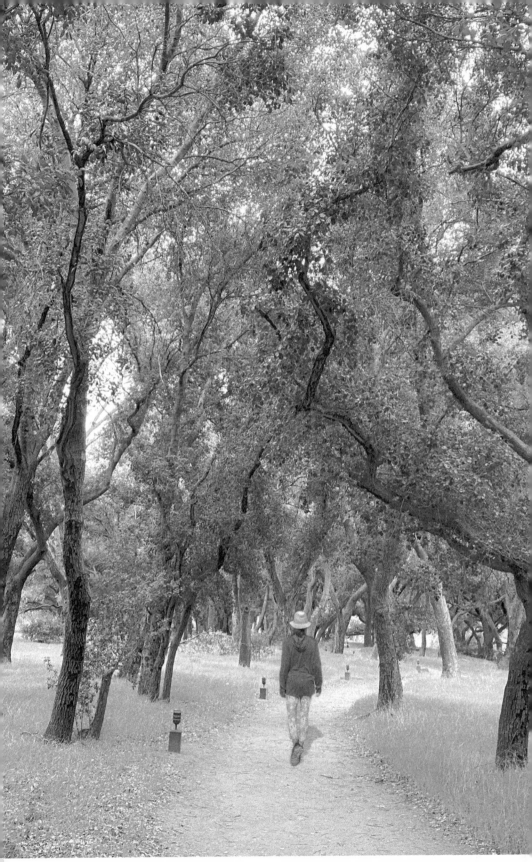

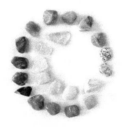

PART 1

My Personal Journey

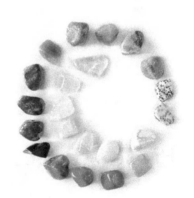

CHAPTER ONE

First Family

By the power of concentration and meditation you can direct the inexhaustible power of your mind to accomplish what you desire and to guard every door against failure.

– PARAMAHANSA YOGANANDA

*E*ach of us picks our family before we are born. It is a complicated process that we do with our unseen team of helpers, such as angels, spirit guides, and family members who have passed away. We do so for a variety of reasons, one of which is to nurture our inbred talents. In some instances we may follow in the footsteps of gifted family members. But often things are not as straightforward as that. We might pick families that trigger us into directions that otherwise never would have been possible. For example, having an alcoholic or abusive parent could lead one to heal oneself and then to enter a field of healing. Suffering a deep family trauma might enable someone to teach others about that particular situation, since the trauma itself was a teacher that uplifted their awareness. Life is so complex that many of us experience all the above or any number of variations and combinations. Most important, we are here to grow, expand, and experience more of our unlimited multidimensional selves. Nevertheless, our family of origin is where our earthly story begins.

I was born into a typical middle-class family in the late 1950s, sharing my mother's womb with a twin. I have a distant memory of wanting to get out fast; I made sure I was born ahead of my brother. I had a sister two years older than me who I worshipped. A true creative artist, she was the ringleader in our sibling band, and her word was law—until our mother weighed in. Our mother, a beautiful and cultured dancer and model, was the queen of the household, and what she said was the law. My dad was the benevolent king who only wanted to make peace with everyone. My mother raged and was angry with us a lot, but we adored and worshiped her nonetheless.

By the time I turned eleven, our insular world had expanded. My sister had her own group of friends, and I had a best friend, Cheryl, who I hung out with all the time. That year was pivotal in so many ways. For one thing, it was the year leading up to Woodstock, not long after the dawning of the Age of Aquarius, which was a turning point on the planet.

In late 1968 I was trying to figure out my own life, and the changes in the world at large, when my dad came home one day and told us our mother had cancer. I had no idea what that word meant, but it turned our lives upside down.

Mom was in and out of the hospital for at least three months. One night I cried myself to sleep. I understood with a deep inner knowing that even though my dad said she would be fine, she would not be anything of the sort. Four months after that, in February 1969, my wonderful cousin Marsha and my dad sat my siblings and me down to tell us our mother had died. That moment was the turning point in my life. The three of us were completely grief-stricken. Our mother was our rock. I had always imagined I would grow up and live next door to her, but now I knew that day would never come.

Our dad did his best to hold the family together, but it was so difficult for him to work full-time and make meals for us, let alone supervise our homework and outside activities. Thank God for Maggie, our full-time housekeeper. A five-foot-two African-American ball of fire, she had been with us since my brother and I were born. (Out of stress, I would put all my dirty clothes under my bed, and she would find them and raise her voice in her Southern accent, "Laurriee, get those clothes out from under your bed!" I would giggle, knowing that her raised voice signaled that she loved me.) Thank God, too, for Lucky. That was our family hybrid dog, a friend that I cherished. She was also a safety net for me.

Going back to school after my mother passed away, I felt like a stranger in a strange land. Now all the other girls had mothers and I didn't. It was the first time I started to experience envy, and my mental state was dim and getting darker. I didn't have any tools to pull myself out of the deep valley I found myself in, but I tried to stay positive for my twin brother's sake. My sister pulled away from me, though, and we argued about everything. We all needed so much help, but we didn't get it until many years later.

Within a year, my dad began to date and met a woman named Janet. I thought she was really pretty, and she was very kind to us. Janet had two sons from another marriage. Before long, she and my father wed. Within one year's time, my mother died, my dad remarried, our family expanded, and we moved from the Woodmoor area of Baltimore to Randallstown, Maryland. It was only thirty minutes away, but it felt like a world away from my aunt, uncle, cousins, and anything familiar. Any semblance of normalcy and security were stripped away. Eventually I would remember who I am beyond my physical earthly family, but it would take me decades. All I knew right then was that this was the scariest time of my life. Everything was unfamiliar and I was terrified. What had most rooted me in a sense of security was my father, and now he was taken up with this new marriage and with my two new inherited brothers. I tried to keep up appearances, but I was so unhappy inside.

The greater issue underlying my unhappiness was that my mom's death became a taboo topic of conversation in my family. Because my father and *bonus* mom wanted to move on as if nothing had happened, the trauma deepened inside and I felt there was no safe place to vent. My brother, sister, and I had no tools to process the trauma. It became a dark secret that didn't rear its head until many years later at the Rancho La Puerta health spa and beyond. I was so young when my mother died—my mother, my link to all of life—I was devastated. No outer remedy could heal this wound. No amount of boyfriends, drugs, or drinking could take the pain away. My mom and dad were caring, loving people, but they had no idea what to do with three children who were deeply wounded on many levels.

I went to a brand-new school and, by mistake, was put in a slow class, where I was determined to get A's. At first I had no interest in making friends with anyone. However, by the end of the year, I did start to make friends, and this turned out to be really important to me—in fact, more important than anything. I became friends with Debbie, who was edgy, voluptuous, and popular with the boys. She came from a broken home like me, and what I think I liked most about her was that she was willing to try anything to get attention.

That summer, Debbie and I routinely sneaked out at night and hitchhiked thirty minutes away to another town to meet up with some other kids from school. We got into every drug that was out there, smoked cigarettes, and drank anything alcoholic we could get our hands on. We hung out with, and lay down with boys that were strangers. We were quite a mess! I know I was being protected because, despite my recklessness, nothing irrevocably bad ever happened to me that summer. It's amazing that I survived. It took me many years to realize that my angels wanted me to live.

The following year I went off to high school while Debbie remained in junior high. I resolved to quit smoking cigarettes, quit all forms of drugs, straighten myself out, and leave the friendship behind. I somehow got myself to focus on school over the years and was even cast in some theatrical productions in my senior year. It was the best year of my entire school life. I became best friends with Carol, and her family more or less adopted me. They were kind and caring in so many ways. I went boating with them, had wonderful meals at their house, and felt like I was completely accepted. They were in many ways my Earth angels who loved and supported me with so much of the kindness and nurturing I desperately craved. In 2020 Carol's mom passed on, and I realize now how much she was a role model for me in my life. She will be missed greatly.

Underneath, however, I was depressed and angry about my life and even had suicidal thoughts. Nobody in my family knew it, and as one of five children all struggling for something, I felt unseen. In fact, my family life was in turmoil. I couldn't get along with my new mom, whom I was told to call Mom, and my sister and I fought all the time while having nothing to do with our brothers. Little did I know that I would come to adore them. I can't blame anyone. My mom was probably trying to keep it together with all of us as she worked full-time as an elementary school teacher and had dinner on the table seven nights a week along with packing lunches for five children. My dad worked full-time as a chemist and helped us with homework at night. Luckily we still had Maggie, and she was my rock in life. We rarely had deep conversations, but she had known me since birth and I knew she loved me. But for her and Steve, my twin, I felt completely alienated and alone in my own home.

Life began to change when I enrolled in some ballet classes. I wasn't very good, but I loved the focus and concentration that ballet demanded. By the end of each class, it seemed as though my problems had disappeared. After attending a few different colleges, I enrolled at Maryland's Towson State University for a dance degree. I also was accepted into a small modern dance company that I worked really hard to audition for. I loved the experience, relished my new friends, and admired our director, who inspired me and believed in me. We gave many concerts and performances. My depression was still lurking, but dancing became a form of meditation and therapy.

After that year, I decided I would leave Baltimore once I graduated college and go to New York City to dance with the best teachers on the planet. I knew I wouldn't be a professional, but I still wanted to learn from the best teachers, which became a theme throughout my life. I went to the city in 1981 with another great friend, and we rented a small apartment together. The country was in a bad recession, and I searched all over for employment, finally landing a waitressing job. I took classes at a cool modern jazz studio in Greenwich Village. I loved the classes and the deep concentration they required. While studying dance, I also found a studio that offered yoga classes. I became very interested in yoga because I thought maybe this could be a way to find happiness and pull myself out of my depression once and for all.

I left New York for a summer when I was invited to join a small dance troupe in Boulder, Colorado. While there I read my first metaphysical book: *Out on a Limb* by Shirley MacLaine. I loved every bit of it, and it started me down the road to spirituality. The renowned actress opened the doors beyond religion to her own metaphysical self. The book completely intrigued me, and I began to wonder about my own spiritual journey, which I was clueless about at the time.

Somehow, throughout my depression, I always had a boyfriend. They were my Band-Aids. I moved in with a few of them during my years in New York. One of them, John, I married in 1986. He was charming, eighteen years older, and absolutely infatuated with me. I am fairly sure I was looking for a father figure in John. We had very little money. He was trying to get his construction company going, but at every turn he made big mistakes in his business.

We borrowed money from someone who was a good friend at the time, and my husband went right through it as though it were water gushing from a faucet. That faucet dried up, and after three years of going nowhere in this marriage and continually arguing about how to get out of debt, I was beside myself. I finally broke down and went back to Baltimore to visit my parents.

My mom told me how she left her first husband because he was a gambler. She said her father had advised her to leave him because her life would end up in shambles. That was the best advice she ever gave me. I heard that story and was determined to find a way out of the hole I was buried in. What really inspired me was a little book by Paramahansa Yogananda titled *The Law of Success*. I read it over and over to help give me the confidence I needed to leave my husband and believe in myself.

I returned to New York, where I was teaching dance and aerobics at the time in a wellness center in Nyack, about forty-five minutes north of the city. One day I was looking through my IDEA Health and Fitness Association magazine and found an ad looking for fitness instructors to teach at the world-renowned Golden Door Health Spa in Escondido, California. The name Golden Door rang a bell in my head because the previous summer John and I had shared a house with my friend Susan in the Hamptons, where I taught aerobics at a studio and met a group of women who often talked about this spa. They mentioned it was one of the most exclusive spas in the world. I was intrigued and found the name Golden Door unforgettable.

As soon as I saw that ad for an instructor, I immediately filled out an application for a job interview. I didn't expect a response, but I got one along with an offer to pay for half my flight to California. I agreed to visit the spa and told John I was going away to check out this job—and to have a trial separation. I had no idea how my life would radically change. The night before leaving, I found myself in the bathroom throwing up. I was out of my mind with fear but willing to go forward. The path felt so right and so scary at the same time.

To practice a meditation
that relates to this chapter, visit

meditationsbylaura.com

Access code: **blessings**

click on

WHISPERS FOR RELAXATION
WHISPERS FOR MASTERING FEAR

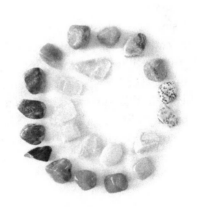

CHAPTER TWO

Heavens on Earth

Be grateful for whoever comes, because each
has been sent as a guide from beyond.

– RUMI

I went first to Los Angeles to visit with my astrologer friend, Spider. He interpreted my first astrology reading, saying that my life would become an earthquake and that I would be going west. He was with my friend William, whom I'd always had a deep crush on (though it never went anywhere). However, I have to admit he was one of the elements that motivated me to travel three thousand miles away from New York. I had never been anywhere except to Florida and back for vacations, and this was the thrill of my life so far. My favorite cousin, Jeff, sent me off with $2,000 as a loan since I had no money to my name—only joint debt with John. I vowed that even if it took me my whole life, I would pay him back every cent.

I rented a car and drove to Escondido, arriving at the world-famous Golden Door Health Spa. I was astonished by the front doors, which were literally gold in color. I walked through these twelve-foot doors to the most exquisite grounds I had ever seen, lush with greenery, trees, and the scent of lavender and eucalyptus. I thought, *This has got to be Heaven. Where else could I possibly be?* I was led to my own small cottage, and someone came to invite me to the most delicious dinner I had ever had. The food was incredibly healthy, colorful, and delectable. Most of the vegetables came from the organic garden that was on-site. I went to bed so happy and content and beyond excited for the next day

I was invited to take all the classes. By the end of the day I was thrilled with everything at this spa. I had a conversation with Judy in Human Resources. She asked me if I had a car and a place to stay. I explained I didn't since I had just left New York for a trial separation from my husband. She suggested that I go down to Mexico for an opportunity to work at the Rancho La Puerta health spa, which was the sister spa to the Golden Door. I eagerly agreed. She called to let them know I would be coming down the next day and arranged for a driver to take me to Tecate, Mexico.

My head was now spinning. I couldn't believe the turn of events. I had another amazing dinner and sleep. I was so excited about this adventure that had presented itself. I had to pinch myself to see if it was real.

The next morning I woke up early because I felt like a kid going on a super amazing vacation. I couldn't stand to sleep any longer. I popped out of bed, dressed, and had a yummy, healthy breakfast. As soon as I finished, a sweet woman led me to the front door where a driver took my one small suitcase.

The driver was wonderful, and we chatted the whole time about Rancho La Puerta. He told me this was a world-class one-of-a-kind spa, and people from all over the world came to it. It was one of the first spas in North America, started by a husband-and-wife team who were committed to people's health and well-being. I was so excited to learn more about this couple, Professor Edmund and Deborah Szekely. Their son Alex was now the managing director of this spa. I couldn't believe I was on my way there for a job!

We drove down through San Diego where I saw the Pacific Ocean for the first time, and I just about dropped my jaw in amazement at its beauty. The weather was eighty degrees, with a warm breeze that caressed my face through the open windows. As we drove farther south toward Mexico, the roads became quiet. The dry landscape—mountains dotted with trees and protruding gray rocks—was like nothing I'd ever seen. I was definitely in the West; there was nothing Eastern about this place.

We drove through a winding, mountainous road to get to Tecate. There were no buildings of any kind—only more mountains, more trees, and, now, giant boulders that looked as though they'd erupted out of the ground. Somehow this was beyond western now; I felt as if we were on another planet. As we headed onto the main road toward Tecate, we saw a small gas station and a convenience store off to the left and a modest market to the right. Then we were at a tiny guard station that demarcated the border. A guard casually signaled us to go through. Welcome to Mexico!

At the time, Tecate was a small town, and as I looked around, I attempted to put my high school and college Spanish to use by deciphering the signs in shop windows. There were bakery shops for dulce y leche—sweets and milk products. There were a few gas stations and open-air clothing stores with shopkeepers sitting out front observing passersby. I didn't see too many Americans walking down the street. Tecate looked more like a town for the locals than a tourist destination. Within five minutes we pulled off the road to approach the Rancho La Puerta health spa. Now I was truly mesmerized.

We drove up to the entrance to the administration building. As in Escondido, I was awestruck by the front doors. But these doors were not golden; they were made with colorful glass and huge forged-iron handles. Once again I felt as if I were entering Heaven. I signed in and was directed to the fitness director, Phyllis Pilgrim. Walking at least half a mile along perfectly manicured, flora-lined walkways was an otherworldly journey. The buildings along the way were typical Spanish architecture, made of stucco with slightly pitched roofs. There were bronze statues of women in meditative or yoga positions. Lavender and rosemary fragrances pervaded the air so much, I imagined I was on the grounds of a perfume factory.

I finally made my way to the staff lounge and met Phyllis. She was a sprightly, energetic woman in her mid-fifties with a strong British accent. I immediately loved her. She said to me point-blank, "I have been praying to the Universe for a dance teacher." I said back point-blank, "That's me. I can be that dance teacher for you." She hired me on the spot.

Apparently, it was difficult to arrange for instructors to come down to Mexico to teach in 1989. I was thrilled beyond words for the opportunity. As Phyllis led me to my room, I continued to be astonished by the grounds—about four thousand scenic acres I was told—spectacular in every way. There were groomed pathways with a diversity of flowers and plants and commanding ancient oak trees, each one with a palpably strong presence. The backdrop to the entire scene was Mount Kuchumaa, a sacred Indian site that reigned over Tecate in stately fashion. I could have happily gone on walking forever.

We walked over a large bridge that led from the realm of guests to the realm of instructors—the area where the staff stayed. We walked down a cement pathway to an area called Motel Row. Its rooms were quite simple and quaint: each had a bed, a refrigerator, a bathroom, a little patio, and oddly, a small television, but it lacked the ability to receive signals from any TV stations. No telephones were in the rooms, although I had noticed a few scattered here and there around the spa. As I soon discovered, it was expensive to make a phone call from the Ranch telephones. The staff usually drove across the border to make calls from phone booths on the California side.

I unpacked my one suitcase and then met with Phyllis in her office to go over my schedule for the week. It was filled with observing and assisting in many of the classes. I wouldn't begin to teach on my own until I was trained in the ways of the Ranch.

As my decision to stay and live at the spa sank in, I realized I had only a single small suitcase filled with clothes—certainly not enough to last for more than a little while. The next day, after more delicious meals and a magnificent sleep, I went to the Mercado, a store on the grounds that sold fitness clothes. I needed clothes to teach in, and I figured I could make this work. I bought enough clothes to last for two weeks of teaching. My days and nights were consumed with a strange juxtaposition: peace and relaxation along with incredibly hard work.

At that time, the Ranch was almost a nunnery. Only half a dozen men worked among many female instructors. There was Raymond, who ran the circuit and weight classes like they were part of military training. Everyone loved Raymond. He was tough but kind. Manuel helped Raymond manage the gym. Steve, gentle, quiet, and sweet, taught a lot of different classes and had a home right over the Mexican border. He had been working there for many years. Joe, another longtime staffer, led bird-watching, hiking, and many classes. Marcos, the lead tennis instructor, was always making jokes, and many times I was taken in by his pranks. I loved them all, including Kurt, who felt like a brother to me and was kind, generous, and also made us laugh.

Among the many female instructors, one of the ones I felt closest with was Michele Hébert, a yoga instructor whose classes I kept finding reasons to take. She was always passing on sage advice she had received from someone named Walt. I didn't know at the time that this Walt was the renowned yogi and spiritual master Yogi Raj Walt Baptiste, one of the key individuals who brought yoga to the west, nor that he would become a big part of my yoga life in years to come. Michele would later become a senior teacher in the Walt Baptiste method of Raja Yoga who guides students to purposeful evolution of consciousness through classes and retreats.

We staff members became a family, replacing, for me, the family I lost when I was a girl. Some instructors rolled in and rolled out; some stayed for a few months and then went on to the Golden Door Spa at Sea program. Rancho La Puerta had contracts to place its instructors on cruise ships around the world, and this was a highly sought-after program since the opportunity to travel, teach, and see the world was attractive and desirable to all of us. Still, many of us stayed together and bonded deeply. The days went by seamlessly, filled with classes, hiking, and quiet time to write and connect with other teachers.

For me, this period was profoundly healing on many levels. For the first time in my life, my stress level dropped significantly. My new friends were funny in addition to being kind and loving. With them, I laughed like I had never laughed in my life. We laughed so hard we had tears in our eyes, on hikes, and virtually every time we did anything together as a team. After dinner, we congregated at each other's tiny casitas and laughed some more.

In this environment, the dark days of my youth, which had weighed so heavily on me, began to fade. One day while hiking I heard a voice, which I knew was an inner voice, address me for the first time in my life. It said, "You have a hole in your stomach area." I knew I didn't have a physical hole but instead an emotional hole that needed to be addressed. I had been journaling in my spare time, and when I journaled about this, I came to understand that my depression covered up a deep sadness about losing my mother. I began to feel safe enough to look beneath my surface to visit with my old companions "pain and loss," who, incredibly, became my dear friends. When they started to appear, I felt safe enough to welcome them as a way to explore, on a deep level, what happened to me and why depression had been my constant companion for so long. My journey inward had begun.

I realized I was still connected with pain and loss over leaving John. He told me one day that he was suicidal when I left, and I felt that deep inside. I felt his hurt whenever I called him. I would cave, hang up, and sob. I knew it wasn't my fault, but it was so hard to hear him aching so much. Even though I described our situation as a trial separation, he was reeling at the possibility that I could leave him permanently. Being at the Ranch was a godsend because John couldn't visit me, nor could he call me daily. I was in a safe, loving environment, able to gradually let him go. However, it was my leaving John that ultimately opened up my core wound—the loss of my mother—which had never been fully addressed.

I was teaching a lot of the fitness and dance classes, and led many hikes in and around the foothills of Mt. Kuchamaa. My confidence grew as I got better and better at the work I loved, and the healing continued. My debts lessened as I was being frugal, even when I went into San Diego on my days off. I was determined to pay back my cousin Jeff. Each week when I received my paycheck, I would send him something to chip away at what

I owed him. I had all my debts and payments posted on a wall, and I would pay him and everyone else slowly but surely.

After about eight months of my living this lifestyle, Phyllis asked me if I wanted to join the fitness staff on the QE2 cruise ship with three other instructors. I was so excited by this opportunity that I again said yes immediately. Michele, who had already worked on cruise ships, gave me yet another piece of advice from the mysterious Walt: use the opportunity to meditate, and to meditate even more at sea than on land. I would try to honor that.

One of the coolest parts of my trip was that we were to board our ship in Baltimore, which meant I got to visit my family. From there, it sailed up to New York City. This was an amazing sequence of events, because it also gave me the opportunity to meet with John and sign formal separation papers with ease and gratitude. Our meeting was platonic and beautiful. John was gracious, and no harsh words were exchanged. He took me back to the ship, and we said good-bye.

I felt really good about the whole experience and knew my life was about to change forever—again. An unseen hand seemed to be purposefully setting up my life as I began more and more to trust my internal guidance. The serendipity of being able to get to Baltimore to see my family and then to New York to take care of the separation papers felt like I was living in the magical flow of life. Abundance was flowing in from everywhere, allowing me to stop worrying and trust that there was a higher divine plan in operation.

The voyage our ship took was called the Trans-Atlantic, which meant it crossed the Atlantic several times and landed in the Bahamas and various Caribbean islands. I was so excited to go to all these places that I didn't think much about crossing the ocean. It turned out to be challenging because I would get seasick and had to find ways to stay quiet and lie down during those phases of rolling ocean waves. Apart from that, we staff members had a blast. The fitness instructors and the massage staff hung out together all the time. We had so much fun dancing, eating, and going ashore to visit local villages and churches.

When our three months were up, I headed back to the States and had a great visit with my sister in Texas before returning to the Ranch. Over the years we grew closer as I became more confident, which helped her to finally accept me. When I arrived at the Ranch, I went to dinner to see all my friends. There was a new instructor there named Stephanie. She and I became best of friends. She was a soul sister, and remains so to this day.

Then a day came that opened doors beyond anything I could have imagined. Alan Herdman from London came to the Ranch along with two other instructors. It was 1990, and Alan led a class on Pilates, something I had never heard of. I was immediately captivated by this work. I saw it as something I could continue doing for the rest of my days. More than anything, I fell in love with Alan as a human being. He was kind, gentle, funny, and seemed like the caring big brother I never had. I took all his classes and hiked with him every day. He invited me to England to study with him for free. His offer stunned me. I immediately went to Phyllis and asked her if I could go and learn from Alan and bring this training back to the Ranch. Phyllis and I had a great relationship. She trusted me and loved my enthusiasm, and I could listen for hours to the droll, amusing stories she recounted in her crisp British accent. She loved my idea and loved Alan. It was agreed!

Well, I was halfway to England in my mind. It brought me back to a time when I told a family member, "I am going to travel the world." And that person said, "I don't think so." I was determined to make my statement a reality and never let anyone tell me I couldn't make something happen. Phyllis went to Alex Szekely, the managing director of the Ranch, and pleaded my case. He not only agreed but offered to pay for half my flight. I was over the moon.

There was, however, one small dilemma: I didn't know anyone in England and I needed a place to live for the summer. Serendipity struck again. One day, not long after Alan's visit, an adorable young man named David came to the Ranch as a guest of one of the instructors. He and I hit it off. We had never laughed as hard as we did with one another. Moreover, he was a hairdresser who lived in London, of all places. I asked David if I could stay with him in his apartment and pay rent. He instantly said yes. My plan was now in motion.

I was beginning to think that Spirit was working in my life to help me move forward on my journey. I started to see serendipity I had never noticed before, probably because I had always been so immersed in stress. It's hard to see your angels or guides working in your life to help you out if you're constantly in a state of anxiety.

Next, I needed work. I couldn't afford to take off a whole summer without pay. I wrote to Alan and he told me not to worry; he could help find something for me when I got to England. I was so close. I even had spending money to start off with.

Back in the late '80s and early '90s, we Ranch instructors got the idea to put our classes on audio cassettes for guests who wanted to "take the Ranch home" with them. No matter what class someone took from me, I was able to provide a recording. They sold like proverbial hotcakes. I'd sold so many cassettes and made so much money, I was nearly out of debt. I knew I still had to find work once I got to England, but I was okay with that. I trusted that a higher plan now operated in my life, and it was very exciting for me. I began to feel a freedom I had never known.

The summer of 1990 I flew to London. The excitement I felt couldn't have been more palpable. It coursed through my veins. I felt like my life was beginning again, in the way it had when I first arrived at Rancho La Puerta. David met me at the airport. We visited Shakespeare's home and surroundings, and then he took me to his family home to visit with his mum and dad. We had tea in the tearoom and a delicious English meal of shepherd's pie and greens. His parents were delightful and kind to me. It was such a pleasure meeting them and hanging with David. We laughed and laughed until we were blue in the face. What did we laugh about? Everything!

After a few days of touring, David took me to his apartment in Camden. Camden was filled with young, edgy-looking people. Dreadlocks, tattoos, and black clothing were ubiquitous.

David's apartment was a small one bedroom with a tiny kitchenette and a little living room with a sliding door leading to an outdoor patio. I looked around and wondered where I was meant to sleep. Well, the floor became my best friend. I wasn't thrilled with the living situation and was determined to find a room to let, as they say in England. I gave myself one month to find a more appealing accommodation—one that included my own bed.

Each day I went off to Alan's studio and took Pilates classes on all his equipment. He welcomed me with open arms, and I reminded him that I still needed to find work to support my being there. He made a phone call, and then said to me, "Go to this studio in Kensington and speak with Sarah. She is taking a leave for the summer and needs a replacement." I practically ran out his door to the tube—the British term for subway. At the Kensington Dance Studio I met with Sarah, and sure enough, she needed someone to replace her three days a week to lead a movement class. I was thrilled and ended up having a blast teaching. I earned so much money from those few classes that it completely paid for the trip.

The highlight of the summer was meeting my new soul friend Nikki and her boyfriend, John. Nikki was also a dancer and took Pilates with Alan. I felt like I had known her all my life, and we became best friends overnight. Our friendship led me to find a new place to live within a month of arriving in London. I was grateful to David but couldn't wait to leave his man cave and find some peace, quiet, and a real bed. My new apartment was the cake; the icing was spending time with Nikki and John.

They took me to Gloucester, where we visited an ancient lighthouse and spent the night in an old cottage near the coast. Another time we drove through the Cotswolds, an area in south-central England with rolling hills rising up from emerald green meadows. A quaint, rural, historical village comprising homes made with Cotswold stone, and perfectly manicured lawns filled with flowers and fruit trees, took my breath away. It was classic historical England at its finest. We took walks and spent time at a lake. It was magical having these two individuals as my new friends. I felt safe, secure, and happy being in London. The summer ended on a high note as I said good-bye to all my new mates and headed back to Rancho La Puerta.

As soon as I returned to the Ranch, I approached Phyllis about starting a new class to integrate all I had learned in London. The Pilates class became so well attended that we expanded it to several days a week. I also kept up with my yoga training with my friend and teacher Michele Hébert. The following November, she invited me to El Salvador for a two-week retreat with her beloved master teacher Walt Baptiste and his wife, Magana, also a most important leader in bringing yoga to the West. I jumped at the opportunity to study with both of them.

I had told Michele my intention was to find my soul mate. She remembered that and reminded me of that intention. Just before leaving for this retreat, a guest at the Ranch who'd gotten to know me a little asked me if I was dating. I said no, and she said she wanted to set me up with a man named Gary, a veterinarian who lived in San Diego and ran and owned a small-animal practice. I loved that he was a vet because I wanted to be one when I was younger but knew that I'd feel awful putting animals to sleep. Gary couldn't call me because we had no phones, so I called him and we decided to set up our first date in January, after the upcoming holidays and my two-week retreat with the Baptistes.

What an amazing two weeks they were. We meditated and did yoga every day with Walt, Magana, and Baron, their eighteen-year-old son. Walt took us into pyramids for absolute "blacked out" meditations where no light entered. We learned many ancient breathing practices that have been passed down through the ages. But we also had time every day to swim in the ocean and to practice walking meditations. It was a life-transforming interlude. My meditations became home for me and awakened a part of me that had been asleep. My intuition and dreams became stronger as I began to sense and know things before they ever happened.

After we returned to the Ranch, I continued to work on my newly developed Pilates classes, which I began to teach to teachers. But I kept on meditating, and my intuition grew stronger with each passing day.

One day in December I was holed up in my room, sick with a fever, when there was a knock on my door. Phyllis walked into my room and said, "I have an offer for you." My eyes lit up as she asked me if I wanted to go on another cruise ship for four months that would travel halfway around the world. Of course! I was slated to go the following February with another instructor, Lynn, and together we would run the fitness, yoga, meditation, and Pilates program. My life was on a roll, and I was determined to go with it. It was truly a time of restoration, preparing me so I would be ready, in years to come, to dispel the dark cloud that was still living inside me.

To practice a meditation
that relates to this chapter, visit

meditationsbylaura.com

Access code: **blessings**

click on
WHISPERS INTO WHITE LIGHT
(for healing and clearing)

CHAPTER THREE

Two Men Sharing My Heart

Love is two waves in the ocean where lines cannot be drawn.

– SWAMI VEDA BHARATI

When January arrived, it was time for my blind date in San Diego with Gary. I was a little resistant that evening; I had a terrible cold and it was raining, so I was a bit nervous about driving over the Tecate Mountains. But my dear friend Carol, who was staying with me, insisted I go. She fixed my hair, lent me her car, and picked out an outfit, so off I went.

I met Gary at a San Diego hotel, where we had tea and appetizers. He definitely was looking me over, and I was checking him out too. The weather outside was getting nasty, with black skies and torrential rains. I was concerned about driving back over the mountains. Gary saw my concern and offered to drive me up to his home in Escondido. I'd just met him and thought, *How can I go to his house?* But after demurring for a while, I finally agreed. I had a good feeling about him but was nervous nonetheless.

We went back to his home, and he was a perfect gentleman. I slept in the guest bedroom (which became our son's room years later) and heard the voice in my head: "You will marry this man." What? I thought I was losing my mind, but the voice was loud and clear. Ever since I'd begun working at the Ranch, my intuition was getting stronger and stronger, and many times I received messages out of the blue. When I heard this, I was too tired to argue with Spirit, but I eventually set up a challenge to question this voice. I would know soon enough if this was the right partner for me. Sleep came fast and morning came early. Gary and I had a great breakfast together with lots of chatting. I had to get going since I had classes to teach that day. We said good-bye without even a handshake.

I had five weeks before leaving on my cruise ship for four months. Gary and I talked by phone, and he came down to the Ranch to visit with me. He fell in love with the Ranch and, I think, with me. For the next four weekends we got together and had an amazing time hiking, talking, and eating delicious meals. It seemed like the start of a wonderful relationship, but I had my doubts. I even chastised myself. "I always pick the wrong guys." In a way, I was blessed because I was going away soon, and this would challenge the two of us to see if we could withstand the separation and still want to see one another on my return.

Gary asked for my itinerary and was determined to stay in touch. The day I was heading out to the ship, he and his friend drove me to the Port of Long Beach. His friend just so happened to be heading in that direction and was happy to take us there. We hugged and said our good-byes. I had such mixed emotions. I was sad to leave him but excited about my adventure.

Once onboard, Lynn and I ran the whole fitness, yoga, and Pilates program. It was one of the greatest opportunities of my life. The ship was built for seven hundred people, and we were at full capacity. It offered a wide variety of entertainment and activities, including shows and all kinds of evening programs. As crew members we had guest privileges. We were treated with great respect and were able to go everywhere and do everything the guests could do.

We sailed to so many places, some of which I had barely even heard of: Singapore, Malaysia, Hong Kong, Tonga, Tahiti, Bora Bora, Australia's Great Barrier Reef, New Zealand, Portugal, Spain, France. Everywhere we went, Lynn and I searched for churches to meditate in, great local food to eat, and beautiful beaches where we could swim in the ocean. We met fascinating people from all over the world. But the most astonishing part of this whole grand adventure was that Gary found a way to get a letter to me in every port. It was beyond my wildest dreams that someone could care that much and put that much effort into keeping in contact. I was smitten and skeptical at the same time. I would go to bed and talk with my angels and ask pleadingly, "Please give me a sign if this is the man I am to be with for the rest of my life." I didn't trust myself at all. I always seemed to attract guys with deep issues and major problems.

One night I had the most vivid dream I'd had in a long time. Gary led me to my parents' house, although it looked nothing like our actual home. There was a swimming pool out front, which in real life we didn't have. Gary hugged me before I left him to enter my home. I heard my sister and mom, Janet, in the back room. I walked back to see them, and they were sobbing. I got very scared and asked, "Why are you crying?" and they said, "Daddy died." I woke up half hysterical. The dream seemed so real I was totally unnerved by it.

We were docked in Dunedin, New Zealand. The phones on the ship would have cost me my whole paycheck, and we didn't have cell phones. I immediately dressed and got off the ship. We were there for one day, and I had to get to a phone booth to call my parents. I walked four miles, passing cows and sheep and feeling like I was on another planet, before I found one. As soon as I saw the phone booth, I ran to it and called my parents. I spoke with my dad first and asked him how he was doing. He said fine. I asked again, "You feel okay?" He said again that he was just fine. Then I got on the phone with my mom, who said the same thing. I was perplexed but relieved. We hung up, and I walked back to the ship.

This was February and I was ending my trip in May. Gary wrote that he was planning a Grand Canyon trip for both of us when I got back. I hadn't connected the dots yet to my dream and, for the time being, wanted to blow the dream off. Losing my mom at such a young age was devastating, and the idea of losing my dad in my mid-thirties was unthinkable.

The trip continued to be a spectacular adventure, and Lynn and I couldn't believe how quickly the time went. When our ship landed back in Long Beach, Gary was waiting for me with open arms. We were so happy to see one another. We immediately drove to his cousin's apartment so I could call my parents again. I was still apprehensive even though it was two and a half months after my dream. I reached my mom, Janet, and she said, "Daddy has terminal cancer." I nearly collapsed.

I started asking a million questions as tears streamed down my face. I hung up and had a huge cry. Then Gary and I drove to the Grand Canyon for the trip he had planned. It was an eight-hour car ride, and the two of us talked nonstop. Gary was empathetic and very concerned about my dad, asking a lot of questions about him. I was able to talk for a long time about my relationship with my dad and how he was a rock in my life. Gary's words were comforting and soothing, but I felt conflicted since I knew I needed to get back to Baltimore to be with my dad. When we arrived, we checked into a hotel and planned our hike down the canyon.

It was the most beautiful hike I had ever taken. The red rocks, deep canyons, and crevices where eagles and raptors hid were astonishing. The Colorado River could be seen as a green line flowing through the canyon in the far distance below. We hiked down to the very bottom and went straight to our campsite and set up a tent. Then we walked to a bridge where we sat and savored a most glorious day. But behind enjoying the stunning views and spending time with Gary, my mind was consumed with my dad.

We lasted one more day there, and then I told Gary I needed to go and be with my father. He was sympathetic and understanding. I called the Ranch to take a leave of absence because I didn't know how long I would be in Baltimore. We hiked out of the canyon and drove to Gary's house where I did laundry and repacked.

I flew to Baltimore, walked into my house, and saw my smiling, adorable father sitting in bed, reading. I ran over to him and hugged him for dear life. We talked about everything under the sun: my trip, Gary, the Ranch, and how he was feeling. I was so happy to be able to be there with him.

Gary and I talked every day, and he decided he wanted to meet my dad. I loved that idea. He flew out within the week, and I picked him up at the airport. We hugged and talked and then drove back to my house. My dad was sitting in a chair at the end of the bed, and Gary grabbed a chair to sit across from him. I was parked on the bed looking at the profiles of the two men I had loved most in this life.

Then the dream came back to me. Gary led me to my home as the man coming into my life; my father was the man leaving my life. My tears started to flow. I realized that my angelic team answered my question in dream form as to whether I was picking the right man for me. I had a deep understanding in that moment that my father was dying, and I needed to accept that fact.

When my dad needed quiet time, Gary and I went into the living room and, for the first time, talked about getting married. For that to happen, I told him I needed to know we could have a child. He had two children from his previous marriage, who lived with him part-time (I had always known that being with Gary was a "package deal"), so having a third child was some-thing he needed to consider. He promised to do so.

He left to go back to San Diego, and I stayed with my mom—who I felt closer with than ever before—for six weeks as my dad went into hospice at their home. After a while I felt like I was los-ing my sanity and needed to get back to the Ranch for grounding. I was so sad to leave my dad but knew I had to. I didn't let myself believe this might be the last time I would ever see him.

I returned to the Ranch in mid-June. I would frequently go over the border to call my dad. The last time I spoke with him was the first week of July. He said, "I have looked in the mirror, and I have accepted my time is up and I know the truth." I bawled my eyes out, but he continued, "Please don't go around crying for me. I want you to be happy." We said we loved one another and hung up, but I was unable to take his advice to heart. I just sat by the telephone booth at the end of the little shopping center at the border and wept for a long time. I didn't know what to do. I had just returned to the Ranch for a few weeks and wasn't sure if I should turn around and go back to Maryland.

Within days of that phone call I got an urgent message to call home. My mom told me Dad died peacefully in a hospice center. I fell apart but somehow managed to plan on going home for the funeral. It was a tumultuous, emotional time because even though I knew Gary and I would be together, my beloved father wouldn't be there for the wedding or to meet his grandchild.

After the funeral my days at the Ranch went by as if I were in a trance, trying to make sense of life. Fortunately, I had an excellent diversion to occupy some of my energies. I had put together a proposal to have Pilates mat classes become an official five-day-a-week program at Rancho La Puerta, and it was given a green light. It became a huge success, and I started training some of the other teachers. It was great for my mental state, having something to focus on other than the loss of my dad.

Gary and I continued to see each other, but I still hadn't met his kids. One weekend he invited me to his house and formally asked me to marry him, agreeing to have a child with me. We talked about my moving in with him in January the following year so I would have time to meet his kids and make sure there was someone at the Ranch who could comfortably take over the Pilates program before I left. An instructor named Cathie was eager to conduct the classes in my place and had actually studied with Alan in London as well. I was relieved to be able to turn the program over to someone who I knew could enthusiastically support it going forward. I felt like I was giving up my "baby," and I definitely had mixed emotions.

I continued working at the Ranch and seeing Gary on weekends. I finally met his kids. In fact, all at once I met his ex-wife, her mother, and both his kids at his son Eric's baseball game. There was a strong reaction of resistance from his daughter, Laura Brook. I could feel her not wanting me in her life and instead wanting it to continue just the way it was: the threesome. Gary, Laura Brook, and Eric were a unit and I was the outsider. I understood in that moment that the romantic bliss I'd experienced over the last three years could possibly disappear and that my spiritual boot camp might be beginning. Indeed, it was!

Then I heard the voice in my head. "The wounds of the past will haunt you until they are healed."

To practice a meditation
that relates to this chapter, visit

meditationsbylaura.com

Access code: **blessings**
click on
WHISPERS FOR HEALING LOVE

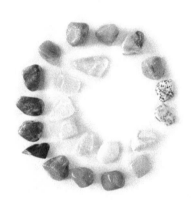

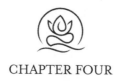

CHAPTER FOUR

Second Family

*Your task is not to seek for love, but merely to seek and find all
the barriers within yourself that you have built against it.*

– RUMI

I moved into Gary's house in February 1992, and from the beginning I felt it was too soon for his kids. They immediately
rebuffed me, and I prayed for a way to become close to them
since I was marrying their father. I didn't yet have the emotional tool set to understand how challenged they were in this circumstance. Their mom and dad navigated this situation as best
as they knew how; still, I was going to be their unwanted *bonus*
mom and all my early wounds from childhood came roaring to
the surface. I was as haunted by feelings of not being wanted, of
being left out, and of feeling as unworthy in this situation as I
was when my dad remarried when I was twelve.

But I was deeply in love with Gary and willing to do anything to make it work. I kept trying everything I could think of
with his children, but what we really needed was straightforward conversation, which rarely happened. The kids suffered
and I suffered, from our wedding preparations onward. I felt I
had some karmic relationship with his daughter—whose name,
ironically, was the same as mine—that needed healing from the
beginning. Her issue was more than thinking I was taking her
father away; she came right out and told me the day before our

wedding that she should be the one marrying her dad, not me. I could see it was going to be a long, hard ride, but since I hadn't done much therapy, I was more or less in an emotional wilderness. Laura and I were both jealous of each other's relationship with Gary. I also knew I really needed to deal with baggage that had nothing to do with her.

My own feelings of unworthiness dated back to my earliest years. I think I had always been envious of my sister, who had immense artistic ability, confidence, and popularity. She always appeared so put together, and never doubted herself. I doubted myself in everything and never felt I was good enough at anything. As the middle child, I was always pining for my sister's attention and working hard to please my mother too. My birth mom was five-foot-ten and strikingly gorgeous. In addition to being a model and dancer, she was an accomplished swimmer, diver, and seamstress, sewing all our clothes. Her personality could charm the world, although there were times when she raged at us if we didn't do things the way she wanted us to. This affected me on many levels, such as my self-confidence and feeling unable to measure up to her standards. Internally this created an intense desire to please her.

Between my mother's and sister's magnetism and talents, and my twin brother, who was quite the outsider in this mix, I was completely lost to myself. The sudden death of my mother exacerbated my alienation. Now, having a daughter reignited all these suppressed feelings. Later, after many years of therapy and spiritual work, I realized she was a mirror for me to look into and view my own deeply wounded reflection.

Fortunately, I was blessed with a new work opportunity around this time. I was invited to start a Pilates program at the Golden Door Health Spa. The Golden Door was close to home in Escondido, so I could have a quick commute or teach privately at home in a Pilates room I had set up. I was amazed at how all this came to be and worked out seamlessly.

Within three months of being married I got pregnant. I was so excited to become a mother to my own child. Gary was thrilled too, but I was worried about bringing a child into our tenuous home life. On top of this, Gary's ex-wife Nancy also became pregnant, so now the kids had two new siblings coming into our delicate and sticky blended family situation. I knew things wouldn't be easy, but I was determined to find a way to make them work. I meditated and kept up my Pilates, which were sources of comfort. The kids were with Gary and me two days each week and every other weekend. We always tried to make their stay entertaining for them. Gary and Nancy definitely put them first, and we tried to keep both households aligned in terms of similar rules and even similar food. But I was really out of my comfort zone and felt like an outsider in my own home. On top of all these changes I was still grieving for my dad.

Less than a year after we married, and while I was still pregnant, I had a most profound dream that changed my life and transformed my grief forever. In the dream, my dad and I were walking down a path by Motel Row, the staff casitas at Rancho La Puerta. He stopped and looked me in the eyes and said, "I am very much alive and at peace. The body is a physical illusion. I am here for you whenever you need me and I love you." I woke up with so much relief and freedom from my grief that I cried myself to sleep with tears of joy. From that night forward, much of my grief around my dad dissipated.

When our son Mitchell was born, I began nursing, which also brought much comfort and healing for me. It was truly bliss for both of us. Gary's kids kept up their visiting routine, but I could tell they weren't thrilled with their new brother, or with me. I tried my best to address their difficulty going between two homes and having two new siblings, but deep down I knew we all needed a lot of therapy to help bring us all together.

By the time my son turned two, I knew our family situation was completely out of my league. I needed help to sort out my emotions and wounds. I found the most amazing therapist, Pam, who I worked with for many years to come.

At the onset of our therapy sessions I had a dream: I was walking around a huge arena, and there was a little person in my pocket. As I walked around the arena I was wondering if I should go farther down into it. When I brought the dream to Pam, we both realized I was walking around my conscious mind and wondering if I was ready to dive down deeper into the unconscious to deal with the loss of my own mother that was buried there. The little person was in my pocket for safety and protection, and that little person was my inner child. Was my little person safe enough to dig down to find my source of healing with this therapist? That was to be determined.

I went to Pam weekly, discovering that my dreams were helping to unravel my deep wounds. My daughter, Laura Brook, continued to be a mirror for me to heal. I also kept returning to Rancho La Puerta, my spiritual home. I went down every year to work with the instructors on new Pilates techniques I had learned. This helped me to continue my own growth and nurture this precious Pilates program I had started. However, the Golden Door was struggling and needed to let go of all its extra programs, including yoga and Pilates, which meant they had to let go of me.

As my therapy continued, one dream in particular was revealing and healing on many levels: I dreamed that I killed my birth mom. Through much discussion with Pam, I understood that I had been holding on to the thought that I was responsible for my mom's death. Pam was so nurturing and loving as I sobbed my heart out. She explained that most people never dive down far enough to get to the source of profound pain, and she wanted me to take this slowly. But clearly there were unseen helpers—my guides or angels, maybe even my mom—wanting me to get through this to the other side for healing.

In yet another dream I was with my mom: We walked into a cancer support group, and everyone started applauding. I realized I was cancer-free and they were clapping for me, and maybe my mom too. But the dream was actually about the progress I was making in therapy.

Then, in the same dream, my mom took me to my life review, as if I had died and was assessing my time on Earth. This is the dream I mentioned at the beginning of the introduction to this book, in which she said to me, "It is a blessing to be alive, and to be in the physical body." That dream was riveting emotionally, mentally, and spiritually in every way and made me realize I needed to practice gratitude and acknowledge all the blessings in my life. I was still emotionally unsteady, but my sessions and dreams were helping me to delve into the stories of my past. I healed a bit more each time I saw Pam.

Dreams became so fascinating to me in how they can reveal our profound unconscious mind and promote healing when we dreamers begin to pay attention. I was so intrigued with this entire healing process that I entered an Energy Medicine program at Holos University, with Dr. Norman Shealy as director. Dr. Shealy is a neurosurgeon and pioneer in pain management and was the first physician to present acupuncture at Stanford University in the 1960s.

I went to his orientation class in Missouri, bringing along my resume detailing my education and years of experience since he wanted to have students be able to enter the master's or PhD program. Taking into account my bachelor's degree and all my outside training, Dr. Shealy wanted me to enter the PhD program with the caveat that I do research and complete a few other courses. I took one course, but the workload was overwhelming, what with being a young mom of a five-year-old and two other young children. So I dropped out. However, it wasn't a waste of my time. I learned so much in the orientation and that one class, and what I learned led me to the crystal bowls years later.

As Gary's kids entered their teenage years, they decided to live with their mom and *bonus* dad full time rather than half the time with us because it was easier for them to be in one place as they juggled school, activities, and social life. Their mom and dad were wonderful parents. Although challenging at times we all worked together to raise happy and well adjusted kids. It was clear Laura Brook still had difficulty with me and never wanted to let me in, let alone allow me to be her friend. I accepted this, but it was hard on me because my own wounds had not fully healed. She was a continual reminder of the loss of my own mother, who I wouldn't see again in this life. An astrologer said to me that I needed to become my own mother. I was working hard on that one. Journaling, seeing Pam, tracking my dreams, meditating, and reveling in Gary's continued love and support all helped.

I continued teaching Pilates, and we moved to a new home that had a downstairs space perfect for teaching my classes and private lessons. As Mitch grew, I decided I wanted to lead day-long retreats and use the tools I had learned over the years to enhance them. I led them for about a year until Gary and I realized that having retreats at our home could create a legal liability issue.

It was about that time, in 2008, that Dr. Mehrad Nazari, a modern yogi who believes in preserving the authenticity of the ancient practices and applying them to our daily lives, and my old friend Michele Hébert told me that there would be a special opportunity at the Ranch to study with an Indian spiritual adept named Swami Veda Bharati. A brilliant man who could converse in seventeen languages, he was officially called Mahamandaleshwara Swami Veda Bharati, a title that has been bestowed on only sixteen of India's spiritual masters. (The Mahamandaleshwars of the Niranjani Akhara are the most learned masters, still passing on esoteric knowledge, composing their own philosophical Sanskrit texts, establishing and guiding institutions, and maintaining financial support for the facilities of their monastic order.)

Using everyday terminology in his discourses, Swami Veda was considered one of the greatest swamis of all time in India. At the Ranch, he would be leading an ashram program running in tandem with all the usual Ranch classes for over a month. It would be an international event with more than ten additional swamis lecturing. I was so blessed because I was already planning to be at the Ranch teaching as a guest presenter for Pilates. I ended up staying for two weeks and went to as many of the ashram's programs as I could.

One day a woman named Ragani was conducting a *kirtan*, group devotional chants, as she accompanied herself on her harmonium—a modified version of a reed organ. She maintained that chanting was "the back door to enlightenment." I was agog when I heard that claim, which really resonated with me, and fell in love with chanting on the spot. When I chanted with her and the group, I felt blissful. It lifted me out of the thin layer of depression that still enveloped me. Someone next to me said, "You will be leading chants one day." I thought, *No, that will never happen.* Years later, it did.

After this experience I started to feel a need to learn more about intuition because of the continuous messages I received in my dreams. I signed up for trainings with a well-known teacher and learned so much about intuition, and about connecting with our angels and guides. As I took her courses, I met amazing people from around the world. Many of them had been trained in Reiki. I didn't know what that was but I was determined to find out.

I researched this method of energetic healing and decided I needed Reiki training. I found a friend of a friend who taught it in Encinitas, California, and proceeded to train with her on Levels One and Two. Between the intuition courses, yoga, meditation, and Reiki, I was, in my own way, getting a degree in metaphysics and energy medicine. I was opening up to a whole new way of thinking about energy, medicine, and vibration. This work, too, was a perfect transition into my practice of healing with sound vibration years later.

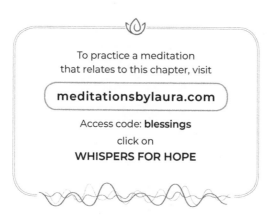

To practice a meditation
that relates to this chapter, visit

meditationsbylaura.com

Access code: **blessings**

click on

WHISPERS FOR HOPE

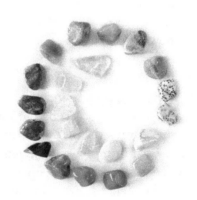

CHAPTER FIVE

Singing Bowls

Sound Healing has been called the medicine of the future.

– EDGAR CAYCE

*I*t is astonishing how fast children grow. Our son was soon to graduate high school and go off to college, and I was sinking into a funk thinking about what was next in my life. Once he left, I desperately wanted to find a path for myself since I was feeling the empty nest syndrome.

Dr. Mehrad Nazari and Michele Hébert were leading yoga teacher trainings and suggested I take their upcoming course. But I felt torn about where, or if, to get such training. I'd always loved Michele and Mehrad and even accompanied them to India in 2011 for a ten-day Yoga Nidra conference at Swami Rama's ashram, Swami Rama Sadhaka Grama, in Rishikesh, India. The ashram was situated near the sacred river Ganga in the foothills of the Himalayan mountains. When we entered the ashram, I noticed a sign—Love, Serve, Remember. Mehrad recently reminded me of that sign. My life is about love, serving others, and remembering who I am, and then sharing it!

While in India I had some amazing transformational experiences. I never dreamed I would be leading Yoga Nidra, an ancient conscious relaxation practice, but over the years I have found it to be one of the most healing practices in all of yoga. I will forever be grateful to Michele Hébert and Mehrad for their exquisite wisdom and teachings from different sacred lineages in yoga and other mindfulness meditation practices. Truly they are luminaries in the world of meditation and are devoted to raising consciousness on the planet.

According to Swami Veda Bharati, Yoga Nidra is a state of consciousness for healing. More profoundly, his teacher, Swami Rama, stated that, beyond relaxation, it is positive preparation for death or "conscious dying." With much practice, we can learn to liberate the soul from the body, conquer fears relating to death, and transition into death with great ease. It is immeasurably valuable to enable dying to take place gracefully and peacefully, as opposed to passing away in a fear-ridden state.

Beyond learning to prepare for death through this deep practice, we bring ourselves into what is referred to in modern psychology as a "hypnagogic state," a state of consciousness that is between wakefulness and sleep but not quite either. This state of mind is exceptionally receptive, and much can be learned quickly in this state—for example, learning to remove unwanted habits.

Beyond such behavioral purposes, as Swami Satyananda Saraswati writes in his book *Yoga Nidra,* "[The practice] can be used for directing the mind to accomplish anything." It can lead us toward our greatest inspirations and unleash intuition by opening the "third eye" and taking us beyond our personalities into the realm of divine consciousness. With an exquisitely still mind, we can access our true nature: pure, authentic, unified consciousness comprising the entire universe. With this access, we can move beyond our three-dimensional self toward our multidimensional self.

Even though I had such a profound experience with Michele and Mehrad in India, I wasn't sure their course was the right direction for me even though it was my idea for them to hold this training.. This perplexed me because of my relationship with them. But I was beginning to learn to listen to my intuition more, and I had my doubts.

The night before I was to give Mehrad an answer, I had another revealing dream. I heard a voice that said, "You don't need any more training." It was clear and loud, and I asked, "Who are you?" and I heard, "God." I literally jumped in bed when I heard that word. It was obvious that my guides had another direction for me, and I took it to mean that if I needed any further training, it wouldn't be with Michele and Mehrad at this time, though I loved them dearly. I prayed for their understanding and trusted that it wouldn't affect our friendship.

In the following months I read about a yoga training at a studio in Encinitas. Intrigued, I began to attend classes and fell in love with the place. I learned that a five-hundred-hour training was being offered there a few months later, and for whatever reason, it felt right in my gut. The training was wonderful, but the most profound part was my connection with Tony, who helped lead the trainings, and his wife Marcia, who taught classes in a form of yoga called Kundalini—an esoteric discipline meant to channel the powerful "coiled serpent" energy at the base of the spine and incorporated these interesting crystal bowls in the final resting pose. I felt a deep bond with both of them.

I had been studying there for a while when one day Marcia asked me to substitute for her hatha yoga class. I would be fine with the yoga part, I knew, but I was unfamiliar with these crystal bowls she played at the end of each class. I had no understanding of how to play them or what their significance was but their soundstook my breath away. I asked her how to play them and she said, "Oh, you just go around like this, running the wand around the rims to make these sounds." I thought, *That seems kind of weird, but I think I can handle five minutes of this.*

I subbed for her class and played the bowls. I had no idea what I was doing, but I fell in love with creating the sounds. After class I knew I had to get a set of these bowls. I ordered them and began experimenting. As I got more proficient, I found out the studio was beginning to offer classes twice a month called Sound Healing Night. I became fast friends with Grace, the woman who was leading the sessions.

One day Grace invited me to play the bowls with several other players at the studio as part of a Sound Healing Night. It was the most extraordinary experience. At least four of us were playing our bowls in different areas of a large room, and Grace added a gong, a flute, and other instruments to create an ambiance for deep relaxation. Sound healing has become more common now, but at the time no one else was doing this in yoga studios. Fifty to seventy-five people started attending our sound healing sessions. Flossie, the director of the two-hundred-hour gentle hatha yoga teachers' training, started conducting "How to Play the Bowls" classes, which became all the rage.

I continued my playing, and although I still hadn't had any formal training, I began to offer my own sound healing classes out of my home and consistently attracted up to ten students, which was a lot for my small studio. I also had the opportunity to play my bowls at a party at my naturopath's office. While there in a small part of the office away from the party, my big, frosted heart chakra bowl cracked down the center, and I was devastated. After reflecting on what happened, I realized that my playing louder and louder to be heard above the laughter and talking in the other room was simply my ego wanting to be heard—a great lesson for my pride. I learned later that humility is the path to venture on when playing these bowls. Luckily, I'd only had that bowl for a week, so the company sent me a new one. But that was the second bowl I had broken. Clearly I still needed instruction.

To further my yoga metaphysical training, I decided to study with Barbara Martin, who had written at least five books pertaining to meditations with different color rays and how they affect our etheric and auric bodies—the energy field around our physical bodies. I studied with her for three years. During that time, each of her students had an opportunity to have a private session with her. Barbara had been clairvoyant and clairaudient as a child, and now, as an eighty-year-old, had honed her ability to channel higher realms. She would receive clear information that made her seem like she was psychic, but she would never claim that because she felt that psychics could be infiltrated with negative energies. Instead, she used the word "channel" and conducted many protective exercises to bring only beings of light and their wisdom to assist her clients on their spiritual paths.

In my session with her, the main question I asked was why my daughter disliked me so much. Barbara said I had been a mean mother to Laura Brook in a past life, and she still had an unconscious memory of it and was resentful. I was stunned. I knew I needed to work on myself to heal our relationship.

I meditated on a pink ray of light that I brought down to myself and then visualized it going to my daughter, as I learned from Barbara. The pink ray is the ray of love, compassion, and forgiveness. I knew this lifetime was the time to clear my karma and heal because we were ascending as a planet. I began my meditations daily, working with the pink ray. It took a few years to begin to feel a shift with Laura Brook, but eventually I got to the point where I believed she didn't dislike me anymore. Even when she was closer to neutral, I knew progress was possible. (See the Forgiveness Meditation on page 110 for the meditation I practiced.)

In 2014 life rapidly got even more interesting. My husband got an offer to sell his thriving veterinary practice and retire. He was burnt out, our son was in college, and his other two children were well into their late twenties and trying to figure out their lives. Gary looked at me and said, "There's an RV for sale. Want to travel around the country and see national parks?" I jumped out of my skin, eager for a change and ready to leave Escondido. We saw the RV and practically bought it on the spot. It was eighteen years old and a great little home on wheels—compact, cute, and fun. Of course, we had a lot to learn, because neither one of us had ever traveled in one of these vehicles.

After six weeks of traveling we decided to upgrade our RV to a bigger one. We'd also decided to put our home on the market, so we had a lot to do before we left on another trip. Our Realtor asked us to make a number of renovations before selling. We hired a contractor friend, Noel, to complete the work while we traveled.

Within four months we were ready to take off on our road trip. It was a very strange feeling knowing we would be homeless soon, but we were thrilled for the adventure. I told Gary I wanted to go to Mount Shasta, a potentially active volcano at the southern end of the Cascade Range in Siskiyou County, California, and off we went. While there, I found my way to a few sound healing classes and then discovered a store called The Crystal Room, Crystal Tones at Mount Shasta. Gary and I went to the back of the shop, where there were more than three hundred bowls. Store attendant Bev led us through an amazing sound journey for over an hour and a half. I was smitten with the vast collection of crystal bowls sold there. I had saved up my own money and bought my first set of three alchemy crystal bowls.

I still hadn't had any formal training, but I continued to play my bowls while traveling and offered to play them whenever I was in a city or town and stopped at a yoga studio. Everyone welcomed me with open arms, and I played the bowls during *savasana*—the supine resting pose that closes every yoga class. This was more than seven years ago, and not many people knew about the bowls and what they could do. Whenever I played them, I experienced a sense of peace I rarely felt before in my life.

We traveled to many states and national parks throughout the US, taking time to visit our kids, Mitch, Laura, and Eric, and family and friends scattered around the country, including some I hadn't seen in years. We were also making new friends and given opportunities to offer sound healing sessions everywhere we went.

While in Alabama I met some wonderful women who worked with a group called Grandmothers Speak. They actually make contact with grandmothers in another dimension. Sharon McErlane, the original leader of this group, met these grandmothers one day and started meditating with them daily. She brought three books containing deep wisdom into existence. These books clearly show our connection to an unseen realm and prove that we are never alone. We have a team of guides, angels, and other beings who only want the best for us and who nudge us toward the direction of our highest potential in this lifetime.

The grandmothers talked about the imbalances on our planet and how we have gotten too far in the yang direction of competition, greed, and disrespect for our Earth. These spirit guides explain how we need to come back into balance with the planet but, more important, with ourselves. Women specifically need to remember to come home to themselves and move back toward their yin nature, which is the nature of receiving. This nature is receptive to the spirit world and not just our three-dimensional world. We are meant to connect daily with our unseen team through meditation and nature and by allowing ourselves to receive messages that support our daily work in this world. We were never meant to live on Earth without support from above. Since we have gotten so far out of balance, it is women who need to remember their true nature; then men will follow. Then the violence will forever end. Sharon's books are all about our intuitive nature. When women remember that they are highly intuitive and learn to trust that intuition, the world will revert to its original nature: a place of connection and love.

We traveled up and down the entire east coast visiting family, playing my bowls wherever possible, and landing in Boston to see our son. After Boston we went to New York State to visit my friend Stephanie from our Rancho La Puerta days, now a licensed PhD in Ayurvedic medicine and acupuncture. While staying with her for a few days, I received a call from my friend Grace who led the bowl playing at the studio in Encinitas. She said, "You won't believe this. Dr. Mitchell Gaynor is going to be at a sound healing and vibration retreat in New York."

Dr. Gaynor was a famous oncologist in New York who'd learned how to meditate, do yoga, and play the alchemy crystal bowls for his patients. I knew him as the author of a profound book titled *The Healing Power of Sound*, which I had read many times to understand how powerful and useful sound vibrations can be for healing. Any person who played the singing bowls knew about Dr. Gaynor. What were the chances of my being in New York less than two hours away and having the time to sign up for a weekend retreat on sound vibration and healing? Bingo! Grace and I decided to meet there.

Gary drove me to the Menla retreat center where I planned to stay for the entire four-day length of the workshop. It was a most remarkable retreat. All the participants spent only one entire day with Dr. Gaynor, who, after this weekend, would start a book tour for his new bestseller *The Gene Therapy Plan*. Grace and I had lunch with him and peppered him with questions. We were blessed to have spent that time with him. He and I had so much in common that I felt I was destined to meet him. His name even combined my dad's name and my son's name. His son was a few years younger than my son and heading off to college. Most significant, his mother died from cancer when he was young, as did mine. He'd had to deal with that same inner turmoil.

Dr. Gaynor became one of the pioneers in sound healing more than twenty years ago. I can only imagine that the medical community viewed him as though he'd lost some degree of sanity because of the unconventional complementary modalities he incorporated into his practice. Instead, he actually gained a lot of sanity and so did his patients, who were incredibly blessed to have had him as their oncologist.

He approached every client as a healer and listened to their stories. Then he put together a game plan that included Western medicine as well as helping them to find their voice through their soul song and meditation. He realized that most of his clients had some inner turmoil that had never been resolved, and he helped them come home to themselves by enabling them to regain their voices and articulating their unresolved emotions. He gave each patient tools, such as coming up with a song meant only for them. He also played the crystal bowls so they could feel that deep state of relaxation and connection to the sounds of the Earth.

One story that featured prominently in his learning about crystal bowls came from Odsal, a Tibetan monk who, while only in his thirties, developed cardiomyopathy, a rare life-threatening disease that causes enlargement of the heart and usually results in congestive heart failure. He was led to Dr. Gaynor for treatment at a New York City hospital. Dr. Gaynor treated him with traditional Western medicine protocols that included an array of medical tests. But Dr. Gaynor also subscribed to the beliefs of mind-body scientists, who maintain that the emotions affect the body's physiology. This philosophy is inherent in some yoga traditions, which state, "The issues are in the tissues."

Dr. Gaynor was keen to hear Odsal's story. When Odsal was a young boy, his family fled Tibet after the Chinese invasion. They endured great poverty while exiled in India. His parents could barely feed the children, and out of sheer desire to keep them alive, they placed the two boys in an orphanage with Tibetan monks. The parents would visit the children once a year. It was devastating for the boys to see their parents and then have to say good-bye year after year.

During Odsal's treatments, Dr. Gaynor led him through guided meditations, and Odsal shared with him the Tibetan singing bowl. The first time Dr. Gaynor heard Odsal play the bowl, the clamor of New York virtually disappeared. He sat there crying tears of joy, feeling a oneness with the universe in a way he had never experienced before. As they continued to work together, Dr. Gaynor realized that Odsal's disease was lodged in a place much deeper than any treatment could reach. Despite all his medical intervention, he couldn't heal Odsal's broken heart.

As sad as this story is, it led Dr. Gaynor to become—in addition to being a doctor—a therapist and truly one of the greatest healers in his field. He wrote, "It would not be an exaggeration to say that the synergistic effect of the singing bowls and voice tones, when used in combination with meditation and guided imagery, has revolutionized my practice. Indeed, I believe that sound, the most underutilized and least appreciated mind-body tool, should become a part of every healer's medical bag." He also made it clear we are all here on Earth for a reason. Once we realize what that reason is, he said, we need to remember it and then teach it.

What does remembering our dharma, our life purpose, have to do with sound? Everything. When we are in touch with our life purpose and act on it, we bring balance into our lives. When we are not aware of our life purpose, we are disconnected from some part of ourselves, and that can cause an imbalance to our body's natural Circadian rhythms. When we are connected to a higher plan, we tend to flow more with a natural rhythm through life and therefore feel more balanced.

As I learned, everything in the universe vibrates and makes sound. The whole universe is living, breathing, and teeming with life. Within any life form, there is sound or vibration—a sound current. As humans, we live in this sound current. This means every organ, gland, and cell in our body vibrates. We generate our own organic symphonies. Especially since we are made of 70–80 percent water, sound can easily vibrate to a cellular level. We have seven energy centers (chakras) within our body and more outside our body. Each center vibrates at a certain frequency. If any parts of our bodies are out of balance or in distress, that imbalance can become illness or disease.

Over and over at the retreat, Dr. Gaynor explained that healing is a state of coming into balance, harmony, and eventually fulfillment of our dharma or life purpose, which can all evolve together. We are preprogrammed to be able to self-heal. When we use the principles of resonance, we can reharmonize our cells, tissues, and organs that have been imprinted with discordant frequencies. What this means is that when we hear or feel frequencies that literally match the chakras, then we can bring balance back into our bodies. Healing on all levels of consciousness includes the physical, emotional, intellectual, and spiritual.

An ancient form of sound healing is music therapy, which has been around for thousands of years. Pythagoras used sound frequencies for emotional and physical healing. Hathor priestesses in Egypt used sound to connect with the cosmos. For eons, yogis have chanted sacred sounds, called mantras, and used sound for connection. Our bodies are similar to musical instruments that need to be tuned and balanced.

Our discussions led to the alchemy bowls, and I was committed and excited to learn more about them. They all are digitally tested to match the frequencies of our chakras and bring us back into balance. As Dr. Gaynor so profoundly explained, when we allow ourselves deep relaxation, the body can begin to heal. The alchemy crystal bowls have the ability to bring us into the deepest state of relaxation because the tones are primordial in nature. This means these tones can assist the brainwaves to become attuned to the electromagnetic frequencies of the Earth. This attunement helps us to come home to ourselves, which is when healing naturally begins. In Dr. Gaynor's Healing Power of Sound, he writes, "We simply need to become attuned to the very delicate vibrations of the universe, because once we resonate with our true essence, we cannot help but become more loving, more intuitive, more capable of reacting from our most open and compassionate self."

I was thrilled with all this information and the time we spent with Dr. Gaynor. I asked him about bringing bowls into hospitals, and he felt that most hospitals weren't open to that yet, but suggested I could bring them into a yoga class at a hospital.

That weekend was a profound life-changing experience that included some of the greatest sound healers from around the world. One of them, Richard Rudis, a deeply spiritual man who had mastered the gong, taught us about it and gave us a full "gong bath" that induced me into my deepest sleep ever. We also trained with John Beaulieu, who was renowned for his use of tuning forks. Many other excellent instructors led us throughout the weekend, and we learned an enormous amount about sound, vibration, and ancient wisdom. However, I had yet to learn about bowl technique and how to play correctly so I would stop breaking bowls. Somehow I managed to break three classic frosted bowls before I got my real training.

By the end of the retreat, I could see why Edgar Cayce, known as the sleeping prophet and psychic, called sound healing "the medicine of the future." I realized this would be the direction of medicine in the New Age.

More than ever now on our planet, we need to find balance and inner peace daily. Chaos has stepped up in our outer world more than ever before. There is no stability. Our stability needs to come from within. I left the retreat fully inspired and overjoyed to continue teaching and leading sound baths wherever I was called to offer them.

A few months after the retreat, Grace called to tell me Dr. Gaynor had died. We utterly disbelieved that he'd taken his own life, but that is what was being reported. We were in complete shock. I can only pray and hope we find out the full truth about his death one day. This wonderful man was definitely my motivation for ultimately bringing sound healing bowls into cancer centers and hospice services.

After getting back to San Diego to complete the sale of our house, we traveled on to Sedona, Arizona. I attended a yoga studio there, and the wonderful owner allowed me play my bowls at her studio. We stayed for quite a long time in Sedona in our RV. While there I enrolled in a weekend sound healing training with Dr. Dream, well-known for conducting healing with three hundred thirty-three Tibetan bowls. To get to the workshop at a ranch in Washington State, I had to rent a car after my flight and drive for an hour and a half down a long, dark dirt road in the country. But the journey was worth it. The weekend was incredible.

A private session with Dr. Dream was one of the best healing sessions I ever had. He asked me what my biggest challenge was. I answered, with utmost sincerity, "Healing my inner child from the loss of my mother." That came up so fast I wasn't even aware that was going to be my reply. Afterward, my stomach started really hurting. I don't usually get stomachaches, but this was bad. I thought I should go to the Sound Bath that night and maybe I would feel better.

Dr. Dream placed bowls on our stomachs, but my stomach ached even more throughout the whole session. I left to go back to my room. I was so uncomfortable for several hours that I lay down by the toilet in case I needed to throw up. Well, I did, and it was a mess. In the middle of the night I ended up cleaning my mess and the entire bathroom. It took a while, but I felt 100 percent better. I showered and headed to bed, feeling like I'd released so much mental and emotional baggage.

I flew back to Arizona and started searching for more classes to further my sound healing training since I still wanted specific, practical tips on playing the bowls. That's when I found Ashana, one of the pioneers of playing the bowls and a revered instructor in the fields of sound vibration, voice, and sound bowl healing. With a background in singing, she has many CDs highlighting her riveting voice. Her five-day retreat at Mt. Shasta was called Crystal Bowl Mastery. I jumped on it, determined to learn from the best. I had finally found what I was looking for. I learned everything I needed to learn, and more, to expand my sound healing sessions and move on to the next level of playing and healing. Along the way, my bowls were calling me to chant with them. My throat chakra opened up and I found my voice.

Gary and I hit the road again and traveled to Durango, Colorado. But I was getting antsy and ready to settle down; we had been on the road for two and half years. So we considered settling there.

I decided to get a reading with an astrocartographer to determine the best location to live, considering my astrological chart. The astrologer graded different areas around the country, but it turned out Durango was a D for me and would be very challenging. I asked about Montana, Idaho, San Diego—all rated C. He told me the best places to live would be Nashville or Knoxville, Tennessee; Louisville, Kentucky; Minneapolis; and Asheville, North Carolina. Sedona rated a B for me and might be a little challenging. There were sweet spots closer to Flagstaff, but I was okay with challenge, and Gary and I both adored this place and could definitely see it as home for us—maybe not forever but for a while. One consideration was that we needed to be close enough to Gary's then ninety-six-year-old mom and his kids in San Diego, and Sedona was only a six-hour drive. Gary said I had 51 percent of the vote on where we lived, and he had 49 percent. I was quite happy with this arrangement.

In December 2016 we were living in an RV park in Sedona, and I was teaching yoga and leading some sound healing classes. We were hiking daily and loving life. I said a prayer that if we were meant to live in Sedona, I would be given a sign. The astrologer had said that sometimes it's too difficult to live in the A-rated places and people from those areas would come to you instead. He gave me the example of him living in Minneapolis. Ireland was the best place for him but not his wife. He ended up attracting a whole group of Irish friends naturally. Ireland had come to him.

At the end of December 2016 I met Lee Ann and immediately liked her. I asked where she was from, and she said Louisville, Kentucky. My eyes lit up: Could that be a sign? The next day I led a class and met a sweet woman from Knoxville, Tennessee. Two of my A places had sent me emissaries. I thought, *Hmmm... getting interesting.*

We found a Realtor, and I prayed to the Universe. I believed if we were supposed to live here, we would find a home on a particular street, with a casita, that backed up to national forest land. We searched for several months. Everything was either too expensive or needed too much remodeling. There were also several houses without *great bones.*

I decided to take the initiative and start looking myself. Within a few days a new house popped up on Zillow, and I called our Realtor. "I found our home." I just knew it. It was on the street where we wanted to live, bordered the national forest, and had a cottage on the property. I told Gary this was *the* house, and we made an appointment to look at it. The price was less than anything we'd looked at, though it needed complete remodeling. Despite that, Gary and I knew this was our home. We made an offer, and it was accepted. Within two months, the place was ours. We moved into the cottage while we remodeled the house, but even in the cottage we felt we had so much space since we had been living in an RV for so long. It was a feeling of freedom.

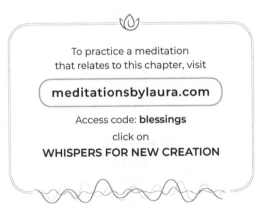

To practice a meditation
that relates to this chapter, visit

meditationsbylaura.com

Access code: **blessings**
click on
WHISPERS FOR NEW CREATION

CHAPTER SIX

Guidance

Out beyond ideas of wrongdoing and right-doing there is a field.
I'll meet you there.

– RUMI

I went to yoga classes daily. I grew close to the owner of the studio, and I began conducting sound healing classes, which were becoming a huge hit for her studio. I took an entire training in Kundalini yoga with her—one of the most profound healing trainings I have ever undertaken. Kundalini yoga was brought to the West because the yogis knew we would need a form of yoga that included mantra, mudras (symbolic hand gestures that direct the flow of energy in the body), chanting, and meditation. This ancient technology was brought down for the Aquarian Age. It was meant for this time on the planet when chaos would reign and we would need stability within ourselves. Otherwise our nervous systems could become unbalanced from all the time many of us spend on computers and technology and not enough time in nature.

I learned that when you can dig down into your second chakra—seat of the emotional body, and of sensuality and creativity—and bring up your core wounds, healing can really begin. I had already done a great deal of work around my second chakra, but this training brought up an old belief system that needed deeper healing.

One day when I was doing my personal kriya—a series of poses aimed at a specific result—I heard the words "I am not seen or heard." I realized deep down that this was a core belief I had adapted to in my life. I thought about it and understood I had always been in the shadows of my sister and also my mother before she passed away. I felt neither seen nor heard. I never realized that this was an underlying conditioned belief I'd bought into. This yoga was helping me to unravel conditioned beliefs about myself. I also understood that this sort of core belief is pervasive in our society in minority groups and in the collective consciousness. Many people feel neither seen nor heard. It was time to break the chains of that kind of conditioned thinking.

Our conditioned beliefs become like a song stuck in our heads that plays over and over unless we substitute other thoughts. We are not our thoughts or beliefs, but we think we are because they become so ingrained. From Kundalini yoga and all my years of yoga with Michele Hébert, I learned to change my thoughts with mantra. A mantra is a Sanskrit phrase that is said repeatedly in order to change negative and positive thought forms to neutral. The power of mantra cannot be overstated. Sanskrit and Hebrew are the two languages that have come down from higher dimensions to facilitate our spiritual growth. I grew up with Hebrew, but Sanskrit was a whole new world. I fell in love with mantra and chanting and appreciated how it shifted me into a happier level of being. It brought me into bliss similar to that of my time with Ragani when she performed *kirtan* at the Ranch. Chanting has become my happy place, a part of my everyday life, and I am always thrilled to chant with others. I am also now part of a regular *kirtan* group where we lead others in chanting—another prophecy that has come to pass.

That year I continued to grow by leaps and bounds. I took a course in something called the Human Design System. Human Design, which combines astrology, chakra study, and Kabbalah, led me to understand why I love teaching and inspiring people with rhythm, music, dance, and song. It was clearly in my chart. There is a right and left profile. If you have a left profile in your chart, it means you are here to teach others about themselves. If you have a right profile, it means you are here to learn about yourself. Neither one is superior to the other. My left profile explained why I love to inspire and uplift people and look for positive solutions. It also showed that my talents were related to rhythm and ideas, which is why I love dance, yoga, and movement.

When you grow up without your birth mom, you don't know who you truly are. That is why I have gravitated to teaching and learning for almost forty years. Teaching gave me clarity about my dharma—my way of and reason for living. Most of us are brought up to get a job that will support us. I wanted so much more than just to survive. I wanted to feel passion and to thrive and to offer that to people I encountered along my path. Human Design was another major tool for me and helped me to understand myself and my family. Funnily enough, my daughter and I have the same profile. We have a unique connection and similar paths.

My training has never ceased. As I prepared for the workshops and courses in Sedona, I started an online course with Jonathan Goldman and took time to read all of his books. Jonathan has been a pioneer in the field of sound healing for more than thirty-five years. I was most impressed with his book *The Humming Effect: Sound Healing for Health and Happiness*. It was such a powerful read, helping me to understand the effects of humming on the parasympathetic nervous system. He discusses how humming alone can be one of the most beneficial things we can do for soothing ourselves, for relaxing our vocal cords, and for healing and transforming ourselves. This literally helped me to open more to my own healing process. There are so many benefits to humming that I began to do it daily. It reminded me when my son was a baby and I would soothe him by humming, rocking, and singing. Really, it was amazingly soothing to me. This new learning gave me a whole new addition to my classes and upcoming workshops.

I also took an Enneagram course that revealed to all of us students our shadow sides as well as the imbalances in our personalities when we are not in our center. I now knew I had not been in my center for nearly my entire life, and this explained my passion for finding balance. This course brought home the importance of what the great William Shakespeare wrote: "To thine own self be true."

When we can learn about our shadow side, healing can happen overnight because we are no longer blinded by dysfunctional behaviors that run us without our even knowing it. These dysfunctional behaviors are our addictions. It doesn't matter whether we have an addiction to people pleasing, drinking, drugs, or even to building thick walls to keep people at a distance. These addictions prevent us from knowing our shadow side and keep us in the dark as to why we keep repeating certain behaviors. I was a huge people pleaser because I never felt safe or secure. As soon as I started to feel more secure, I learned the power of saying no. Once we have an awareness of our shadow side, light can shine on all parts of ourselves and we can accept that being human is wonderful: the good, the bad, and the ugly.

In December 2017 I returned to Rancho La Puerta. I had a wonderful week but realized I had moved on from teaching Pilates. The next time I went back, in June 2018, I led only sound healing classes, chanting, and meditation. Throughout the year I continued to teach at the Sedona yoga studio, and we developed a beautiful sound healing program that took place every Friday and Sunday night.

One day I heard my Spirit voice say very quietly in my head, "Laura, become a distributor of the bowls." I argued. "Why should I become a distributor? I just want to teach and play the bowls." But I felt that strong nudge inside me and finally gave in. I made the investment and led at least three workshops with the owner of the Sedona studio by my side. The owner was amazed; I saw the look in her eyes and knew she wanted to partner with me to distribute bowls and conduct trainings. I knew inside that I would have to leave the studio if I didn't partner with her. And I wasn't ready to leave the studio.

We became partners, and for more than seven months we led workshops and trainings together. But by June I started to get a weird feeling about our business partnership. I loved my colleague, but I felt it would never be an equal partnership because the studio was her baby. I always felt I was in her shadow, even though I had brought the bowls and some of the trainings to the studio. Yet I was still absolutely committed to making our partnership work.

Then I had a dream in June 2019 in which the owner said to me, "Are you going to divorce Gary?" I told her the dream the next day. It scared me because I knew the power of my dreams. I didn't realize at first that it meant leaving her. I had no real conscious reason to break up the partnership with her at the time. We were doing well leading classes together and selling bowls. It was working, but I had a strange, uncomfortable gut feeling. I know she began to feel me pulling away, even though I had no specific reason other than a vague need to find my own path.

Around that time in June, my friend Laura Gideon and I planned to go back to the Ranch and lead classes. I decided it was time to bring along Gary's daughter, Laura Brook. We laughed so hard about being the three Lauras. My daughter and I had grown a lot closer, and she admitted to disliking me for a long time. We spent a magnificent week together laughing, hiking, and sound healing. It made for an incredibly nurturing time, and I believe it healed both of us in many ways.

When I went back to Sedona in July, I had a series of related dreams, including this one:

> I am somewhere with a kind, sweet man holding me and loving me. I don't recognize him in my dream. I leave and go through a subway and see a big dog lying around. I go to my apartment, and my first husband moves in with my two friends. He sits in a chair and closes his eyes. I am looking for something in his dresser drawers, which are filled with women's clothing. Then I tell my friends I'm leaving at the end of the semester and moving on.

This dream felt profound and telling. The kind man could have been a father figure supporting me and encouraging me to go forward. "Subway" is movement forward, and the dog represented loyalty and companionship. My first husband, John, had a strong personality and represented my then business partner who also had a strong personality. In the dream I said I was leaving at the end of the semester. I ended up leaving the business partnership at the end of 2019. Looking through the drawers represented me looking for myself, and what I might be "wearing" in the new year. Who will I be in the year of 2020—the year of clarity and truth?

In August I had another series of profound dreams, which made me feel my guides were working with me on this transition in my life. Among them was the following:

> *I am with a friend who is pregnant. I want to tell her a dream I had about her waiting to do something. My friend says, "Come with me and see my sisters-in-law." We go down the hall and they are all sitting around a table eating different cakes. I say, "Wait for me, I will be back. Save them for me."*

I felt the dream was about me being pregnant with an idea. I went to meet these new women coming into my life, but I was not ready to have sweet desserts with them. I needed more time.

Also in August, my business partner led a group of us to Alaska for a shamanic retreat. I shared a yurt on the top of a hill with my one of my best friends, Sharon from San Diego, away from everyone else. I felt removed from the rest of the group. The other retreatants grew very close because of their sleeping arrangements. Sharon and I loved hiking up the hill and spending time together. At the same time, I started to feel more distant from my partner.

These stirrings continued to grow in me until I knew I had to make a move soon. My ego wanted me to find blame, but I was maturing beyond the need to cast blame. The higher part of me understood I had a different calling. Spirit was now guiding me rather than my ego directing me. This was a new feeling for me, and I was beginning to trust that something bigger was happening for both of us for our highest good. Beyond this, one day during our retreat I burst into tears and knew I needed to put my mom's death to bed for good, that it was time for complete healing. Wow, so many years later and this came up so fiercely I couldn't ignore it. I knew how to do a releasing ceremony on my own because of all the Native American ceremonies I had attended at the studio, and was determined to perform it when I got home from Alaska.

The other profound thing that happened on the trip was when we went on a boat to go whale watching. During the excursion we got a distress call from another boat: A man had fallen backward, hit his head, and stopped breathing. We arranged to meet that boat and bring the man on board since we had two nurses in our party who could perform CPR. As the nurses administered CPR, whales were jumping in and out of the water all around us.

Some of the women on the boat burst into tears at the sight of this man receiving CPR. Soon, a Coast Guard boat met us and took over the medical intervention until we reached land. When we landed a doctor came on board and declared the man dead. We were all stunned.

I prayed that the whales had been sent to ease the man's transition out of his body. Whales hold all the memories of Earth. They are multidimensional beings that are here to help us accelerate our spiritual growth into more of our own multidimensional selves. Whales' energy can assist us in helping us to remember who we are since they are the record keepers of memories from all lifetimes. Furthermore, they inspire us with their high vibration that naturally uplifts our spirits in their presence. They encourage us to sing our soul song. On that day, they showed up with perfect timing to shift our perspectives from our limited thinking to our more expanded multidimensional thinking.

After my initial shock and grief subsided, I realized that when you are around death in any circumstance, it is a time for letting something pass away in your own life. I was still grappling with that weird feeling about my partnership and had had a few psychic readings encouraging me to go my own way. I was scared to death to say something: My partner had become a mother figure to me, and since I had never individuated from my own mother, I was being called to have that happen now. I needed to "bury" and release my mother at last. I was too young to understand burying my mother when she passed away, but now I was ready. I also needed to individuate from my business partner to gain my new independence and to heal that childhood wound that was still embedded in me even after years of therapy and deep spiritual work. It was time to say good-bye to both women who were so significant in my life, each in their own unique way.

When I returned home from Alaska, one of the first things I did was go outside and dig a big hole. I wrote down everything that bothered me about my birth mom leaving me: my feeling of abandonment, having to grow up without her, lingering anger and sadness. I brought out a picture of her and prayed. Then I crunched up all the papers and placed them in the hole and lit a small contained fire. As the flames transformed the pages to ashes, I prayed for the complete release of any energy still inside me that had remained "stuck" on my mom. I could feel the energy lifting as the fire consumed my pages. I felt a sense of freedom and realized I was also ready to experience freedom from my partner. It was a remarkable feeling. I knew my partner and I would be meeting in the next several weeks, and I would be prepared.

After Alaska, Gary and I took a three-week trip to Eastern Europe. We learned a great deal and experienced the land from a different perspective than we'd ever gained from history books. We felt the energy of the wars, talked to people who'd experienced the trials of communism, and went to museums and the Jewish quarters to learn about the Nazis and their crimes. Prague and Budapest are thriving cities, but we spoke with some of their citizens who still felt they weren't free since their presidents were dictators. Feelings of suppression still inhabited their energy fields.

As we went through the days of biking, exploring, and learning about the culture, I had a renewed understanding that I needed liberation in my own life. Still, I recognized this would be difficult for me. As my dream had foretold, I felt that leaving my partnership was sadly like separating from a best friend. I was apprehensive and worried about my partner's reaction.

While we were traveling in Europe, I had quite a few more revealing dreams to support my decision. One of them was particularly memorable:

> *I am teaching a class for my partner. Hundreds of people are attending. It is a huge room for teaching class, and everyone is paying money. My mom, Janet, takes me to my new bedroom. I tell her I am nervous.*

Teaching is what I do in many capacities. I have to teach. In the dream many people wanted to take my class, which was held in a vast space. Huge opportunity is coming my way. I head to my new bedroom, which is symbolic of going to the womb for security, safety, and comfort. My mom, a female I have grown to adore, led me to my new place of comfort, and it was scary to move into this new place inside myself: a place of support, self-love, and nurturing. It is my bedroom, not shared with anyone else. It is a place I had barely experienced in this lifetime.

After returning from Europe but before I met with my partner, I had this remarkable dream:

> *My dad comes to me and says I should change the setting on his college ring.*

I woke up actually inspired to change the setting and wear my father's ring. I was scheduled to teach a class that day and had a strange feeling nobody would come. However, my friend Joy came. Since nobody else showed up, we decided to go for a hike and agreed to meet at the hiking trail. Two minutes away from the studio I realized my dad's ring was missing. I panicked and called Joy to tell her I was going back to the studio to look for it. I searched all over the studio, but the ring was nowhere to be found. I felt like I was in the Twilight Zone.

I went home and checked everywhere I had been that morning. I have lost many items during my life and usually find them when I pray to my angels for help. I typically get a picture in my head of where the object is. But I was so upset about losing this ring, I couldn't get a signal.

I met Joy for the hike and was quite preoccupied with the ring until our conversation engaged me and I forgot about it for a while. At the end of the hike I went home and searched high and low again, with no luck. I surrendered to the Universe with a prayer: "Dear God and angels, if I am meant to find this ring, please find a way to bring it back to me. If I'm meant to let it go and release the material object, I will and will do so with ease." I felt that prayer strongly in my heart and was able to let the ring go. I was just baffled that my dad came to me in a dream and asked me to change the setting. The answer would eventually come, as you will know from having read my introduction to this book.

One night before my partner and I were to meet, I dreamed I was on a 14-carat-gold dance floor, and my partner and I were doing a dance of separation. Gold is the highest frequency on the planet, so it was being done with a high vibration. I felt comforted by this dream.

When the time came, I told my partner in the kindest words I could find, without any blame, that I needed to go in a different direction. We handled it in the most positive and beautiful way anyone could have handled a separation. I realized we were linked through karma, drawn to each other like magnets, and needed to learn many lessons from one another. The biggest lesson for me was confidence that I could do this on my own in my own way. I was ready and excited about the change. I had taught my partner about the bowls, and she taught me that I needed to start believing in myself.

After we parted, I had this dream:

I am in a house, held captive by a man who is in a bedroom upstairs. I am standing by the front door, frightened as can be. I look upstairs and then at the door bolt. I decide in a second to turn the bolt and open the front door as fast as I can. My captor hears the front door open and runs quickly out of

the bedroom, but I am gone. I run and run into the woods
before he can figure out where to find me.

This was clearly about my fear of leaving my partnership and my courage to to listen to the quiet whispers inside my heart.

In November I had an astrology reading. The astrologer said I had worked with children for many lifetimes and was highly connected to the Earth. She told me I had a book that needed to get self-published right away. She also said that this was my year, that I had worked many lifetimes, and that in this life I was to receive some kind of recognition. I had paid my dues. She repeated emphatically that I needed to get my book out as soon as possible because of the alignments of my stars and planets.

I was stunned. I had been working on a metaphysical book for children, but it wasn't finished and needed a lot of work. I was quite baffled by this urgency and overwhelmed by the idea of getting it done. I once again prayed to the universe: "Dear God and angels, if you want me to get this book done, please find a way in the energies of this new year 2020 to have it be done with grace and ease."

As you already know, events in my own life, messages from Spirit, the arrival of the SARS-CoV-2 virus, and the global time-out mandated by COVID-19 all served to convince me, beyond doubt, that the book I was actually meant to write—for now—is the one you are reading.

But while I was spending my days writing, another event transpired.

My ninety-eight-year-old mother-in law, Sally, was in an assisted living home near our Sedona house, and all ten women living there were in quarantine. During those few weeks Gary and I would talk with his mom from outside her window, using our phones. One night we got a call saying she had fallen out of bed. We drove over immediately, and as we arrived, an ambulance came for her. We followed it to the hospital.

The doctors put Sally on morphine because she had broken her neck, right arm, and shoulder. Within two days she fell into a semicoma. With all these injuries and her having little in reserve and being close to ninety-nine years of age, we realized her life was ending. We decided to bring her home with us and enlist hospice help. Our wonderful hospice nurse, Mary, explained the process of how the body lets go. As sad as it was, it was an amazing process to witness. Mary, who we adore and remain friends with to this day, and her five-time Purple Heart recipient husband, Gerry, assured us that Sally was on her journey home, which made us feel better.

The whole family arrived to be with her, and we spoke to her while she was in a coma, convinced some part of her remained alert. Everyone had an opportunity to say good-bye to Sally and thank her for being a wonderful mother, grandmother, and aunt. We made sure she knew she was loved. I played the crystal bowls for her and that seemed to help calm her down a bit when she was agitated. My friend Maryanne and I led a ceremony to help the process move further along, calling upon Sally's guides, parents, and anyone else who was assisting her. The next day she passed away. It was an honor to help usher her and be present for her rather than have her pass away at a hospital.

It made me think that when we come into the world, it is the result of a journey from another world—the spirit realm, Heaven, or whatever you want to call it. It's a transition from one dimension to another—and the same as when we leave this world. As we watched Sally slip away, I could only think that her fear of dying may have prolonged the process. Nobody knows for sure unless they have gone through a near-death experience. However, a book that hospice gave us, The Eleventh Hour, clearly states that when you can relax, you can let your body go. Relaxation is a big part of the dying process. This was fascinating for me to read since it corroborated what my master yoga teacher, Walt Baptiste, said about how meditation teaches us how to "consciously die." When we learn to relax on a daily basis, we can assist in our own ultimate journey out of our bodies.

What also occurred to me during this process was that our society doesn't discuss death. That creates more fear around the whole transition. It is a natural process to end this life and move on to something else. Everyone has their own beliefs about where we go when we die, but as the great Einstein has said, "Energy cannot be created or destroyed. It can only be changed from one form to another."

Although it is a momentous conversation, at some point in life it would be wonderful to have a discussion with family and friends to dispel fears around dying. The Dalai Lama suggests meditating on life and death every day, and I try to do so—even more so now that Sally has left her body. I believe Sally's passing was a wonderful transition for her, and I am so grateful she was able to be with her children and grandchildren.

After the family left our house, I was ready to dive back into the book. As I continued to write my story, I also began leading guided sound meditations online. I connected with dear old friends serendipitously who guided me toward an editor and indie author strategist.

To practice a meditation
that relates to this chapter, visit

meditationsbylaura.com

Access code: **blessings**

click on

WHISPERS FOR YOUR LIFE PATH

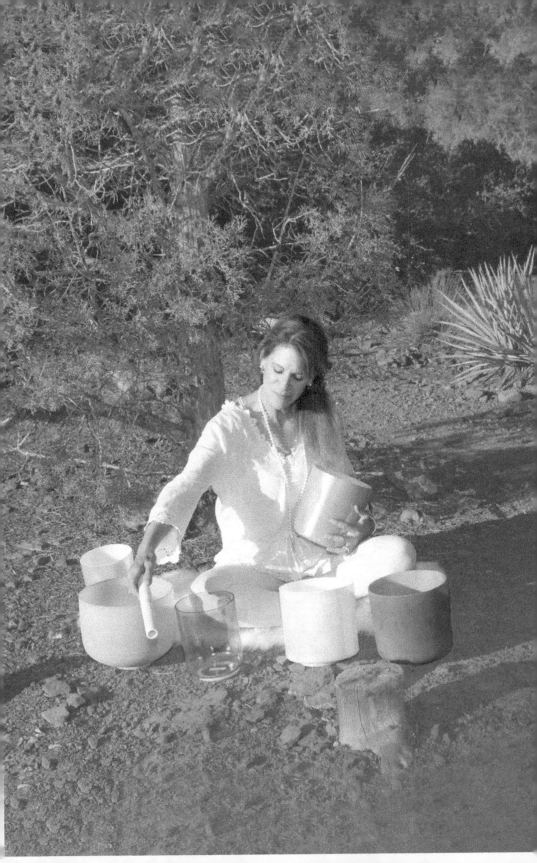

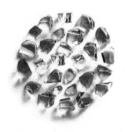

PART 2

Healing Meditations

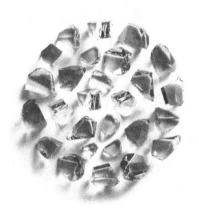

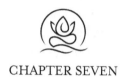

CHAPTER SEVEN

Fast Track to Freedom

*It's your road and yours alone. Others may walk it with you,
but no one can walk it for you.*

– RUMI

So here we all are at the true beginning of a new journey,
moving into a new day and new Earth. This is one of the
most exciting times to be alive. I have felt myself in the shadows
of someone my whole life, and now it is time to come out of the
shadows. I feel tremendous support and know it is time to speak
my truth. I have done so much inner work that I have a better
grasp on the outer world now. We can never go back to the old
paradigm. We are destined to move into a brand-new paradigm
that supports all life on the planet. I am beyond thrilled to be a
part of this whole new world. It is such an opportunity for us to
evolve as a species. I am excited that I can share these meditations that have guided and helped me blossom over the years. It
is our time.

It is Earth's destiny to ascend into lighter and higher dimensions. But dark energies have had a grip on the planet for
thousands of years and don't want to loosen that hold. Among
the dark energies are some corporations who have no concern
for our health and or the health of our planet. They are invested
in pesticides and in pollution from oil and gasoline-powered
cars. Their motivation is money rather than people's well-being,

and they are holding on for dear life. It's sad that the corporations who have caused the most damage have not owned up to what they have done. Pesticides of all kinds have harmed animals, humans, water, and land. Opioids have wreaked havoc, causing addiction and suicide. These are crimes against humanity and must be addressed.

In the future there will be an end to corporations causing illness and death and harming our Earth for money. The new era will use biologic energy, rather than drugs, as the primary source of healing. But I also believe that the barrage of pharmaceutical companies' advertising that nowadays invades our everyday lives when watching TV will be replaced with a belief in what should be a simple mantra, "If I don't make time for my wellness, I will be forced to make time for my illness." We should repeat this simple mantra over and over and allow ourselves to take responsibility for our well-being.

Walt Baptiste always said we are born natural healers and have the ability to heal ourselves. We have gone way off course in allowing pharmaceutical companies to wield that godlike power, undermining our natural ability to heal.

Fortunately, there is so much light pouring onto our planet now that people are waking up everywhere. People are realizing that harming Earth is equal to hurting themselves. There is no separation. We already have technologies that could wean us off oil addiction today. And there are so many technologies ready to be unleashed that can begin to clean up our oceans and land. We are on the edge of a new and astonishing world.

This is also the age to honor the woman. Many ancient prophecies stated that when the women take back their power, the men will fall in line and the violence will end. That means it is time for women to come home to themselves as females and not imitate men. The time for that is ending. The Dalai Lama said, "The world will be saved by the Western Woman."

Thousands of years ago in a land called Lemuria, women were the shamans, healers, nurturers, teachers; they also guided the men to fish by their intuition. The reason is that they carried the sacred seeds of creation within their wombs. These seeds connected to their hearts, and through their hearts they taught the children the ways of the world guided by the moon, Earth, sun cycles, and the cosmos. After many years, the land sank into the seas and the surviving Lemurians carried the sacred seeds of wisdom within their DNA, which was passed down from generation to generation. Over lifetimes, indigenous tribes and ancient cultures held this wisdom of their connection to the cosmos through art, music, sound, study of the stars, and the language of light. Many cultures forgot this sacred knowledge, which led to humans devolving and forgetting their soul reason for being on Earth. However, the shamans, healers, and indigenous tribes kept this knowledge alive for generations.

Through the centuries, it was mostly men who became the leaders of Earth. Women eventually began to learn the ways of man through competition and comparison. They became dissatisfied with life because of the loss of connection to their sacred nature. This tide began to turn about sixty years ago at the beginning of the Aquarian Age. Currently, more women have begun to wake up to their divine nature, remembering who they are and having the courage to share it. Their purpose is similar to that of their sisters in the days of Lemuria: to guide, heal, love, and tap into their intuition. With the resurgence of this ancient dynamic, love and compassion are now rising throughout the land. This is accelerating the evolution of our species. The old paradigm of greed and domination from the Piscean Age is collapsing. The new paradigm of love and compassion is arising.

We are living in the most transformational of days. As I write this, we just experienced the third of three eclipses within a month's time. Eclipses bring in powerful transformational energies that will shake us up and wake us up to more of our true nature. It may feel like we are riding on an emotional roller coaster. We are. We will always remember 2020 as the year of transformation.

The most important message for women is to relax and attract. As they rewire themselves to stop hustling and pushing forward as they have been trained to do, they will remember their true nature. As they relax, they will attract what they need, as they did in days gone by, and they will remember how to employ their intuition in order to receive. Intuition is within everyone, but it is women who still give birth and who understand that deep calling inside to connect with and reinforce the wisdom from the ancients.

The world stopped in March 2020. People slowed down and awakened to what was true for them. People discovered they could work from home and not drive as much, diminishing their gas dependency. It helped people connect through virtual reality so people didn't feel so isolated. People spent more time with their children and in nature. We don't yet have a clue as to how big this awakening is going to be and how it will affect future generations. The Age of Aquarius was just a catchy song in the Broadway musical *Hair* in the 1960s, but it's coming to fruition now and will continue to unfurl over the next ten to thirty years.

I pray with all my heart and soul that I can be around for this incredible show. I pray I can continue to be a channel for anyone who is searching for deeper understanding of the changes that are about to unfold. We truly are in for an awe-inspiring ride. It will take some time since there needs to be a lot of unraveling and cleaning up on the planet. We have disrespected Earth in so many ways, and the destructive residue needs to be reckoned with. We need to begin to heal the Earth and at the same time do our own inner work.

We have come into this life knowing that it would necessitate a huge expansion of our bodies, minds, and souls. We made the choice to be here at this time in history. We are not victims; we chose to come now and learn on the fast track to freedom. As old systems continue to break down, we have to adapt in completely new ways of living. We can never return to materialism as a means of self-esteem. Our self-worth comes from our creativity and from using that creativity in the best possible ways. We aren't meant to be slaves and work only for money; that paradigm is ending. We are meant to shine now on the planet and to use our creativity to overcome fear and anxiety and to open the doors to our intuition. Once you begin to listen to your intuition, you begin to follow your destiny and soul purpose: the new GPS.

That is the new paradigm. The old paradigm will end within the next thirty to forty years, and I applaud anyone who defies its subliminal hypnotic training. We can learn as a society. We have our minds, meditation, nature, healing hands, and sound vibration that can all be used to bring in balance and equanimity.

The most wonderful thing about this time on the planet is our children. The ones being born are so gifted and talented. Some are coming in with no karma: clean, pure slates with no cosmic knots to untie. They are here to use their gifts and talents, just like us. They are coming in to help this whole ascension process happen with greater ease. Their DNA is more activated than ours. It is said that the masters' DNA is completely activated and gives them complete access to their innate wisdom and mastery over time and space. Our DNA is getting more activated now as we become more multidimensional in our three-dimensional bodies. The new babies being born have more gifts and talents than we have ever witnessed before. They will help us to wake up to our higher soul purpose and to realize our own amazing potential for healing.

The energies of love and light are embracing our planet like never before. It is most important to combine these energies with intuition (the new GPS for this Aquarian Age) and to take time every day to find stability within ourselves. To feel at peace, many agree it is necessary to work on it daily. It's an internal job.

Daily chanting, meditation, yoga, crystal bowls, and being in nature all comprise my daily sadhana, my discipline. They are my teachers who enable me to maintain a neutral mind daily and to feel aligned with my infinite nature, my soul. My goal is to practice and experience peace daily, and I know these vibrations go far and wide. I can't fix or change anyone but myself, and after the years of grief and struggle I am finally residing in joy. I am certain life can be and is beautiful. As my mother told me, it is a blessing to be in the body. I feel very blessed to be alive, and I harbor the deepest gratitude to my moms and to all my teachers on this exquisite journey of life. I was told years ago that I needed to become my own mother. That is the journey that has defined my life and now it is time to share that with others.

If my dad were alive, he would ask me, "Laurie, what have you learned?"

I would answer, "'There's no place like home.' I have learned to come home to myself. Nobody could do that for me. Not you, Dad, or my mothers, family, teachers, or friends. You and they were and are my earthly guides. I had to make this journey alone, albeit with a whole team in the unseen realms cheering me along. Thank you, Dad and Mom, for being my support from the other side of the veil. Thanks to my *bonus* mom, Janet, who I think of as simply mom. She's earned it for being my support on the earthly side. I love you all."

This is a new day, a new world, and it all started to blossom when the world stopped. Please enjoy and savor the following meditations. They will help you to access your potential and unleash deep healing capabilities.

We're all just walking each other home.

– RAM DASS

To practice a meditation
that relates to this chapter, visit

meditationsbylaura.com

Access code: **blessings**
click on
WHISPERS FOR A NEW EARTH

CHAPTER EIGHT

Guided Meditations

*T*his chapter of the book consists of guided meditations for facilitating healing and self-love, healing relationships, cultivating inspiration, and healing any harmful emotions not supporting your life journey. We are living in an astonishing era and need to clear out old emotions so we can begin to thrive.

I suggest a crystal for each meditation to help the process move along more quickly. Over the years of workshops, courses, and trainings, I learned a lot about working with them. I have chosen each crystal for qualities and properties that can assist in your transformation. Crystals are part of the Earth, and each one resonates with a certain energy and frequency that can be used for healing and support. They can amplify your intentions, store information, and transform and transfer energy. When our thoughts interact with crystals, they can potentially help our brain frequencies become harmonic and shift our consciousness into higher vibrations. They are powerful tools for renewal and rebirth. If you decide not to work with crystals, the meditations are powerful on their own.

The following crystal-enhanced meditations all begin the same way.

Connecting with Your Crystal

1. Feel the crystal's texture and form and sense its energy.

2. Hold it in front of your face. Blow your breath over it to connect with the crystal and create a relationship with it. Inhale across the crystal and bring its essence into your lungs. Imagine that the stone has accepted your connection.

3. Hold the crystal over your heart. Look down and continue to exhale over the crystal and inhale across it, allowing the energy of the stone to shift into your heart.

4. Continue this breathing and notice if you are feeling any new energies flowing into your heart or your body. Notice if you are feeling a soul connection with this stone, like you are making a new friend.

5. Notice if any images flow into your mind or if feelings of love, inspiration, or joy are being evoked. Notice any physical or emotional shifts in your being. Lastly, notice if you sense any connection to your angelic realm or to the guides who support you. If you aren't experiencing anything, that is completely okay. The effects can be subtle and still help you shift as you continue your practice.

Preparing for Guided Healing Meditations

Please begin by lying down in your most comfortable position with your crystal. If you don't have a crystal, you will still highly benefit from the meditations. Tense your whole body as you inhale. Hold for a few seconds, then exhale and relax your body to release deeply. While exhaling, mentally release anything that is bothering you. Imagine these thoughts flowing out into the universe for healing. Repeat this two more times.

Bring your hands to your heart. Imagine the person who gave you your name. That person loved you so much that they gave you that name, which has significance for you. Honor yourself by saying your name to yourself silently at least three times. Now set a powerful intention for healing of any kind—mental, physical, emotional, or spiritual.

Imagine three layers of light circling around you in a clockwise direction as a bubble of protection, helping to increase your divine light. Rub your hands together for 20–30 seconds to feel warmth and place them anywhere on your body that needs healing. If your feet need healing, hold your hands in that direction to send energy to them. Keep them there as you go through the following relaxation sequence.

Take a long, slow, deep breath for at least 4–6 counts. Hold for a pause on the inhale, and then slowly exhale for 4–6 counts. Continue this slow, deep breathing as you begin to relax your toes, feet, and ankles. Breathe. Feel your legs softening and relaxing. Feel the back of the legs relaxing. Feel the front of the legs relaxing. Soften the hips as you feel them sinking into the floor. Relax your lower belly, mid belly, and all organs and glands in those two areas. Imagine relaxing your digestive organs. Continue by relaxing the heart, thymus gland, and lungs. Feel your heart and chest softening. Go down to your lower back and imagine the lower back relaxing. Breathe. Continue up to your mid back and feel it relaxing. Feel the upper back behind the heart relaxing and softening. Imagine your shoulders dropping down and relaxing the arms and hands. Relax the back of your neck. Feel the muscles relaxing. Feel the neck relaxing. Allow the jaw to relax with the mouth softly parting. Relax the tongue. Relax your face and eyelids. Lastly, relax the forehead.

During your practice of crystal-enhanced meditations, simultaneously listening to the healing sounds of alchemy crystal bowls can help to bring you home to your true self.

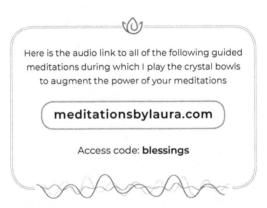

Here is the audio link to all of the following guided meditations during which I play the crystal bowls to augment the power of your meditations

meditationsbylaura.com

Access code: **blessings**

1

Healing Love Meditation, with Rose Quartz

Everyone on the planet needs healing. We have lived through the most challenging times and will continue to be challenged as we grow and expand even more into our unlimited potential.

Place Rose Quartz, a stone with a vibration of pure love, on your heart center. This is a powerful feminine stone of connection to love and to the divine. It supports you in overcoming old sadness and fears. Its love vibrations can penetrate to the cellular level.

Follow the "Preparing for Guided Healing Meditations" instructions on page 93.

With your hands on your body, visualize light radiating from your hands to the area that needs healing. Now imagine the light flowing from your hands being embellished with an energy that pulses on the area that needs healing. Repeat a powerful affirmation such as: *I am healed, whole, and healthy.* Or, *My body heals with love.*

Keep imagining the light from your hands penetrating your skin at the exact location of pain or illness and hold it there for 3–5 minutes. With the power of your mind, tell that area of the body that *it is loved*. Imagine a loved one, friend, or pet to conjure up that feeling of love and direct that feeling into that area of the body.

Pain is how the body speaks to you to ask for attention. Say the words "I love you" over and over, giving it positive attention. Breathe that feeling of love into your hands. Imagine a warmth and love flowing into your hands and into your body. Continue this breathing and speaking love to the area of pain. Allow that area to speak back to you. What is it trying to say? Imagine you are communicating with a child in pain. Give the area a name so you can address it more personally and ask: *What is it you need from me in order to heal?* Keep breathing and repeating those words.

As an alternative to saying "I love you," you can use the Ho'oponopono prayer—a Hawaiian prayer that has strong healing properties. This prayer came through a psychiatrist, Dr. Hew Len, who studied with a shaman in Hawaii. He worked in a challenging clinic for mentally ill criminals who had committed terrible wrongs. It was more like a prison since the patients were kept in shackles. Dr. Len never met with any of the inmates; however, he would look at their pictures and develop inside of himself a deep compassion for them. He assumed they must have been treated horribly to find themselves in such a state. As he prayed this specific prayer with compassion, the inmates started to heal, and over a three-year period most were able to be released and the clinic shut down.

This humbling prayer is most powerful when you can conjure up compassion for yourself and the area of your pain:

I'm sorry, please forgive me, thank you, I love you.

I have used this prayer many times in my life and found it to be incredibly soothing.

Affirmation: *My body heals with love.*

2

New Creation Meditation, with Carnelian

Our thoughts are so powerful. If you can feel your dream or desired creation in your heart, then it is possible for it to manifest. It is your heart's desires combined with your emotions that help bring a dream into reality. If that dream excites you and brings you joy, then you have the ability to make it a reality. Believe that your dreams are possible. The more you can feel it, embrace it, and believe it, the easier it is to come into physical form. The veils between Heaven and Earth are so thin right now that creation can very easily occur.

Many years ago I was training to be a black belt in karate. The test was weeks away, and I had worked hard in my training over a number of years and was ready for the challenge. Yet I was extremely nervous about being able to break two wooden boards. I decided to lie in bed every night before the test and visualize the boards and my heel striking the boards. I would literally feel the sensation in my body. It felt so real; I could feel my adrenaline pumping as I connected to the boards. I could feel the emotional excitement of breaking them as well.

The test day came, and I bowed to my teachers, took a breath, and prayed. I stepped up to the boards and plowed my foot right through them like it was going through butter. I had one more set to break. I stood up to the boards again and with all my might, focus, and strength, I slammed my elbow into the boards, again breaking them like butter. I passed the test with flying colors.

The second chakra is one of the most necessary chakras to heal before we can thrive in our higher chakras. It is the center of all your feelings, emotions, creativity, sexuality, and feeling "good enough." It is the center of creation. Whenever we have been hurt, abused, or wounded, this chakra will need the most healing. Working with the color orange and the quartz Carnelian can help to strengthen this chakra and create balance.

Place Carnelian on your lower belly, below your navel. This crystal stimulates creativity, passion, joy, curiosity, and inspiration. It is a stone that promotes physical vitality, courage, and energy, all of which are needed when you are starting any new project. This quartz will help support you in taking risks and add a zest for life.

Follow the "Preparing for Guided Healing Meditations" instructions on page 93.

Focus on what you are choosing to create:

⬥ Feel it in your heart, breathe deeply, and feel excitement for this new creation.

⬥ Feel it in your stomach and breathe deeply.

⬥ Feel it in your cells and breathe deeply.

⬥ Surround your creation with layers of light.

⬥ Ask your angels and guides to assist you in your creation.

⬥ Thank them for all their help.

⬥ Let go of the details during this meditation and allow your unseen team to take care of them.

Imagine your energy field two feet around you, connecting with your heart and mind. Breathe in divine love and compassion for your own sacred nature.

Affirmation: *My creative ideas [label them] are now being created in my mind and heart. My unseen team is helping me manifest my ideas into physical reality. It is done. Thank you for all your support.*

3

White Light Meditation (Healing and Clearing), with Selenite

White light is sacred. When we work with white light, we can bring in protection, healing, and spiritual connection. It is powerful since it embodies all the colors. It is sacred because it is divine in nature. This divine light has the power to infuse you with energies of higher dimensions, with protection, and with spiritual attunement.

Place Selenite on your forehead. This crystal is fast and effective at clearing the auric field (energy around your body). It supports emotional clearing on all levels and reinforces infusion of spiritual divine light into the entire body. It assists in cellular reattunement for wholeness and healing.

Follow the "Preparing for Guided Healing Meditations" instructions on page 93.

Follow your breath. As you breathe in, imagine a brilliant white light enter into your being; as you breathe out, radiate this light into your surroundings.

Next, breathe this light into your physical body. As you breathe out, exhale any imbalances in your physical body. Keep breathing deeply and slowly.

Now, breathe this light into your auric field. Keep breathing deeply and slowly. As you breathe in, let brilliant white light into your auric field; breathe out and radiate this light in your surroundings.

Now, breathe this light into your mind. As you breathe out, release any old thought patterns such as doubt, fears, and negative thinking. Keep breathing deeply and slowly. Fill your mind with this light.

Once more, breathe brilliant white light into your whole being, and exhale this light into your auric field. Continue long, slow, deep breathing. Envision yourself morphing into a being of light... You are a being of light. See this light spread to the whole planet and see the planet as a being of light... See an end to all suffering and darkness.

Affirmation: *I am a being of light. I am surrounded and protected with divine light.*

4

Meditation for Mastering Fear, with Morganite

One night I had a dream about being with some women one evening. We were testing ourselves to see if we could get past our fears. I saw an alligator coming toward me. I closed my eyes and brought in thoughts of love. I said, "Love, love, love," over and over. In the next instant I was lifted up and the alligator was gone.

Fear is an energy that lives in our world. Some people have more fears than others. Some people will take more risks than others because they feel less fearful. I started taking risks as a teenager and have worked to overcome many fears throughout my life, which has helped tremendously with my confidence.

Place Morganite on your heart. This crystal can help to inspire divine love, which can transform your fears into a deeper connection to your true self. Anytime we connect to our soul self, our fears diminish.

Follow the "Preparing for Guided Healing Meditations" instructions on page 93.

Realize and observe any fear when it arises. Locate where you feel it in your body. Say thank you to the fear as a way to acknowledge it and accept it. Ask the fear what its message is. Perhaps there's an insight in the message.

Now imagine four large crystals of light around you. Imagine these crystals bringing a high vibration of love into your energetic field, dissolving any fears of the past. Send this love frequency as a beam of light down through Mother Earth's core. She will then extend this love back into your being.

Feel the energy of love build within you. Feel it inside you, inside Mother Earth, and at a soul level. You are born from love, and that energy pulses within you. This is your natural state of being.

Fear is not our natural state. Visualize any ties to fear, whether they lie in your mind, emotions, or body... See them being broken down and filled with light. Inhale and accept love, and as you exhale, release all fears. Trust that the fears are being released and replaced with love and acceptance. The Morganite crystal amplifies this field of love, acting as a strong eternal connection to the Creator. Feel peace wash over you as you continue to feel this connection.

Affirmation: *I am love, I am loved, I trust in LOVE. I now align my body, mind, and spirit to the loving light of the Creator. I embody the love of the Creator as I imagine this love pouring through every part of me, cradling me to help me feel secure and loved, and helping to dissolve all feelings of fear. I am filled with love, and trust the divine plan is working for the highest good in my life.*

5

Golden Ray Meditation for Hope, with Citrine

I had a dream about my beautiful loving friend Sunnie from Rancho La Puerta. She is wearing yellow gold clothing and I had yellow gold sheets on my bed. The dream felt so happy and uplifting; filled with hope and optimism for the future.

Currently, many people feel despair or hopelessness because they can't see the bigger picture. The bigger picture is that we are moving from a society of greed and separation to one of unity and compassion. Chaos is necessary to break down old systems in order to introduce new technology and bring into government new people who are committed to making our world a better place.

Place Citrine on your upper belly, above your navel. This crystal stimulates optimism, confidence, creativity, mental clarity, joy, passion, and the ability to manifest. It also works on the second, third, and sixth chakras by opening inner doors to increased mental clarity, and helps spark a vision for the future while generating human will. As a result, hope and optimism are qualities generated by this unique gold-yellow crystal.

Follow the "Preparing for Guided Healing Meditations" instructions on page 93.

Visualize a golden egg in your heart, and see its golden light as the light from infinite creation. Repeat to yourself, "All is in divine harmony." Imagine the golden light from the heart expanding into your entire body. See it expanding into the entire room and extending beyond to the entire Earth. Envision it radiating to the sun. Imagine it traveling to the outer reaches of our galaxy. Energy of the heart merges with the energy behind all creation and imagine the golden ray coming back into your heart. See this golden ray of light expanding out to all of creation.

The energy of Citrine and this golden ray encourages hope, security, safety, and connection to all life. Envision yourself and all people happy, laughing, and filled with joy.

Affirmation: *I fill myself with optimism, joy, and passion for life. I am creative and inspired by my joy for life. I feel hope and joy spreading throughout my whole being and my consciousness.*

6

Forgiveness Meditation, with Lepidolite

Forgiveness has been one of my biggest lessons in this life. I grew up like many people, blaming and feeling angry at others for why my life wasn't working. Through the years I came to understand we are all here to learn lessons. Each person has a unique path and lessons to be learned. I was never taught that we all have a unique journey and we all have different gifts and talents to share. It hurts ourselves more when we hold onto resentment or anger. The best and highest path is learning to forgive all those people who have hurt you and knowing that everyone is doing the best they can to manage their lives. I work on forgiveness daily, and it feels so good to let go of resentment.

Place Lepidolite on your heart. A stone of serenity, this crystal is wonderful for calming frayed nerves. It can help you to take the high road in any challenging situation. Also, it can help dispel harmful emotions and negative thoughts, which can lead you to accepting situations with greater ease and forgiveness.

Follow the "Preparing for Guided Healing Meditations" instructions on page 93.

Envision yourself in the most beautiful surroundings. See and feel every detail of that place. Feel the air, see the vivid colors of the surrounding area, see what you are wearing. Smell the different smells, and most important, notice how you feel.

See yourself surrounded by a few people who love you unconditionally and feel their love shining into your heart. Feel their complete acceptance of you and how nurtured you feel in their presence.

Bring to your mind someone who has been a challenge for you in your life. Imagine that person in front of you and try to see what they have been through in their life and why they are such a challenge. Try to step into their shoes and understand on a deep level their personal suffering. Everyone comes into this life with something they need to work out and work through. If you can understand on a deeper level why they are difficult for you, then you can find compassion. Ask your higher self for assistance in forgiving yourself first and then in forgiving that person for anything they have done that may have hurt you.

Envision a pink ray of light extending from yourself to that person. See this pink light surrounding you and then surrounding that person. This color has the energy of compassion, love, and forgiveness. See this ray of light extending between the two of you. Imagine a powerful healing taking place without ever speaking any words.

Allow the energy of the pink ray to work for you, and ask your guides to help clear up any misunderstanding between you and the other person. You don't need to worry anymore; everything is in the hands of your unseen team. This is when you can completely let go and relax.

Affirmation: *I allow myself to release all anger, frustration, and disappointment toward anyone in my life. I allow myself to release all grudges. I forgive myself for anything I have done unconsciously that may have hurt me or anyone else. I forgive anyone who has hurt me and trust that we are all doing the best we can in any given situation.*

7

Meditation to Heighten Your Intuition, with Sodalite

Our intuition is our connection to that still small voice inside that guides us. It is our internal compass. It shows up as a gut feeling or strong visual image in your mind, in a dream, or in your environment. It may show up as a great idea when you're driving, in the shower, walking, or anytime you're relaxed. We get messages all the time, and when we learn to listen, hear, or pay attention, life seems to be more in a flow. For example, one day when I was driving in San Diego and talking with my friend on the phone, she was wondering if she should move to Las Vegas. In that very moment, a truck drove by with big letters on the side that said LAS VEGAS. I thought there was no way that could have been a coincidence. It felt like a sign from the Universe. She did move, and it was the best step for her. I truly believe that when we pay attention to the signs around us, we become more aligned with our natural flow and attuned to our life's path.

We are living in days of chaos and inquiry. Many of us are questioning everything in our world. Stability in the outside world seems impossible to find. We are being called to find our own inner stability. Homing in on our inner resources and intuition is necessary to withstand the pressures of change and the unknown. As we strengthen this ability, we become our own best teachers and guides.

Sodalite is a stone that can enhance your intuition and insight by its connection to the third eye. It can assist you in connecting to the world of spirit. It is an excellent stone for assisting with discernment and seeing beyond the five senses.

Place this crystal on your third eye. The deep blue color and the properties of Sodalite will help to open your intuition and deepen your ability to connect to your higher self and beyond.

Follow the "Preparing for Guided Healing Meditations" instructions on page 93.

Breathe the energy of blue throughout your body. Set an intention to awaken your consciousness. Envision your third eye below the center and in the middle of your forehead, behind your eyebrows. Allow yourself to open that eye to infinite wisdom and your own innate divine intelligence. Breathe into that darkness and relax into that space of peace. Allow any messages to come through and write them down if necessary.

Affirmation: *I am highly intuitive and trust my intuitive nature. I allow myself to open to my own innate divine intelligence.*

8

New Earth Meditation, with Labradorite

As we step further into the Age of Aquarius, chaos abounds to dismantle the energies of the old paradigm. Where our attention goes, energy flows. Instead of focusing on the old world collapsing, focus on the new world you would like to envision. This meditation leads you into a positive, optimistic vision of the New Earth. Focusing on a new vision is highly empowering and beneficial for all our senses and our well-being.

Labradorite is a stone of magic, adventure, and travel into the inner realms of your Self. With your intention, your outer world can be transformed with the aid of this magical stone.

Place Labradorite on your third eye. Breathe deeply into this powerful crystal of transformation, and imagine a future filled with optimism and hope.

Follow the "Preparing for Guided Healing Meditations" instructions on page 93.

Imagine yourself walking through a forest as you feel the ground beneath your feet. Feel the energy of the Earth pulsing through your feet and legs. Feel the energy in the forest as you notice the trees swaying in the breeze and the wind on your face. Notice the sun shining through the trees and the leaves glimmering in the light.

You meet with a grandfather and grandmother who hold the wisdom of the ages within them. They lead you to a glimmering bridge—a bridge engulfed in all the colors of a rainbow. The bridge is filled with purple, blue, yellow, pink, orange, red, and green colors weaving in and around the bridge. You cross over the bridge with your grandfather and grandmother. As you walk over the bridge, you feel a strong energetic pull of joy and peace. When you reach the other side, you see people joyously dancing under the midday sun. The air is fresh, clear, and sparkling in the sunshine. There is a joyous feeling in the air. As you continue to walk forward, you notice the Earth pulsing and vibrating with life. The ground feels alive.

You continue down a path to the ocean. Dolphins playfully jump in and out of the water with their big whale brothers and sisters by their side. Imagine two dolphins jumping out of the water to kiss you on each cheek. Notice how pure and clean the waters are; you can see clear down to the bottom of the ocean. Beyond the ocean you see mountains that are pristine in their regal stance. You lift up on a cloud with your esteemed companions and travel around the Earth to view its beauty and purity. The rainforests are teeming with life. The trees are vibrating brightly with energy, and the animals are happily roaming around. As you shift your attention to the rivers and streams, you notice the same clarity and purity in their nature.

You head to nearby schools and walk into classrooms filled with children learning by using all their senses and excitedly learning new skills. The teachers share wisdom with joy, and the children are content and happy to learn in an integrated multidimensional way.

You lift back up onto the cloud and soar over to the nearest hospital. The hospitals are now wellness centers that help bring people back into balance and healing on all levels. As you enter, vibrant colors and smells of aromatherapy and plants fill the surrounding areas. There are windows that draw in the sunlight for healing, along with crystals embedded in the walls. In the center of every room are beds lined in crystals to bring in balance and recalibration. Doctors and nurses are assisting people to become well and whole. Chemotherapy and drugs are a thing of the past. These centers are designed for rebalancing and recalibration.

You smile at your beloved guides. You climb back onto your cloud with them, and it takes you back to the rainbow bridge. You realize your journey is to assist you in expanding your vision and intention for the New Earth. You feel joyous and filled with optimism and hope knowing that we are indeed becoming a new world.

Affirmation: *I am filled with optimism and joy knowing we are heading into a New Earth filled with endless possibilities of love, joy, and peace.*

9

"Waterfall of Peace" Meditation, with Amazonite

I love waterfalls and have one outside my home. It is so sooth-ing and peaceful to hear. If you can imagine a waterfall flowing through your body, the visualization can bring in much peace.

Amazonite is a stone that generates harmony within yourself and others. It is the great peacemaker. It can help you to speak the truth without being overly emotional and to feel peaceful before speaking. It can also magnify any intentions of healing difficult relationships.

Place Amazonite on your heart. Its turquoise blue color is very soothing to the throat chakra, and the properties of this crys-tal will calm you and allow the energies of peace to enter your heart center.

Follow the "Preparing for Guided Healing Meditations" instruc-tions on page 93.

Imagine a blue light in your heart. This blue light transforms into a waterfall. Imagine this blue waterfall cascading over your heart, thymus gland, lungs, digestive organs, into your muscles, tissues, all organs and glands, down to a cellular level. As the waterfall spreads throughout your whole body, imagine infinite peace, infinite joy, infinite calm, infinite healing, infinite wholeness, and infinite peace.

Affirmation: *I feel at peace, I am filled with peace, I am peace.*

10

Life Path Meditation, with Lapis

Life is meant to be in a flow. We are meant to follow our inner promptings and listen to that still small voice that guides us in many ways toward the highest path in our lives. When I follow my intuition, synchronistic moments happen more frequently and everything in life seems to be flowing with greater ease.

The following meditation can lead you to glide more smoothly on your path while helping you to realize we are never alone. We always have assistance in this world from our unseen team— our guides, deceased loved ones, and angels.

Place Lapis on your third eye. Lapis is a stone of royalty, of visionary awareness that activates both one's third eye and throat chakra for speaking your truth. This stone of inner vision can assist in enhancing your visual images and manifesting your intentions into reality.

Follow the "Preparing for Guided Healing Meditations" instructions on page 93.

Breathe deeply and visualize yourself standing upright and sending a beam of light down from the top of your head to the bottom of your feet and anchor this light beam into Mother Earth. Surround yourself with love flowing from her to you. As you visualize this light beam, imagine your crown chakra opening at the top of your head.

Now, see yourself lying in a boat with cushions underneath you for comfort and support. Feel your emotions and your physical and spiritual bodies perfectly supported. Imagine every detail of this boat. What kind is it? A canoe, rowboat, long boat, sailboat, or motorboat?

Breathe deeply and relax. Imagine the boat is in divine flow as you gently move downstream. You don't need to guide it. The boat is floating in the direction of your soul. Imagine a presence of guides and angels in the boat and all around. They love you and support you. Relax and see if you can visualize them and feel their elevated energies. Hear chirping birds, splashing water, and wind blowing through the trees in the distance.

As you relax more, the boat glides more purposefully in the direction of your soul. A message is downloaded to you from your angelic team as they assist you on your life path. When your boat guides you to shore, you have clarity and an inner knowing of the highest and best direction for your life. You thank your angelic team as you leave the boat.

Affirmation: *I am filled with clarity and renewed direction in my life. I thank my guides and angels for assisting me in my life's path.*

11

Speak Your Truth Meditation, with Aquamarine

I was fortunate enough to study with Wah! She has worked with healing sounds for many years, creating mantra music, healing concerts, and relaxation and meditation music for the yoga world. She has helped pave the way for me in my healing work, as well as trained sound healers around the world. Her work involves toning and connecting our heart to our voice. Because many of us haven't been supported in speaking our truth, this connection brings healing on many levels. Now is the time on the planet to open our throat chakras and speak that truth.

The following meditation assists you in opening the throat chakra and enables you to speak honestly, become a better listener, and communicate with clarity your deepest desires. The throat chakra is called the soul's gate because it links your heart to your head. As you open up the throat chakra, you begin to heal all levels of communication between yourself and others.

Place Aquamarine below your throat, close to your heart. This blue crystal is excellent in assisting you to communicate with greater ease, calm, and clarity in any situation. This stone can help you become effective, clear, and loving in your heartfelt communication.

Follow the "Preparing for Guided Healing Meditations" instructions on page 93.

Begin with deep breathing. As you breathe, take in the translucent blue in your mind's eye. Envision this blue color coming down from above your head into your throat. Continue your deep breathing. Imagine this color in your throat. As you imagine the color or speak the words blue in my throat, repeat the following affirmation. Keep repeating the affirmation many times until you feel its truth in your heart.

Affirmation: *I communicate my truth and desires with ease and grace. I am safe to speak my truth. I listen deeply to those around me. As I envision this color blue in my throat, I am healing any imbalances in my throat and heal all lifetimes of any speaking dysfunction. My throat is now healed from the traumas of the past, present, and future.*

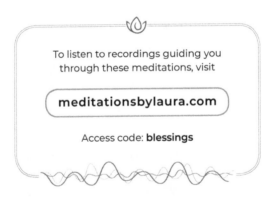

To listen to recordings guiding you through these meditations, visit

meditationsbylaura.com

Access code: **blessings**

Epilogue

I hope and pray these meditations can assist you on your journey. We need tools now more than ever to manage our minds and emotions. Our world will never be the same. We will never forget 2020 as the year when the world stopped.

As we move deeper into the Age of Aquarius, the use of color, sound, and light can be transformational tools to gracefully ease our inner journey into this "Age of Light." Our New GPS is our guide to this new day. If we want our lives to flow with grace and ease, we must remember to listen to this age-old navigation system—our intuition—and tap into the energy of love. We can transform our world into a realm of love and peace

Love is the most powerful force in the universe. It can create stars, planets, and galaxies, as well as our own babies. Women hold that powerful seed of creation inside of them. Men need to soften and learn more about their true nature to find their own unique rhythm and balance to be able to assist in this new world. Now more than ever we need to do whatever we can to uplift and inspire humanity to shift the energies of the planet. We are witnessing the old consciousness falling by the wayside. People are unwilling to accept the lie that we are separate beings. We are all connected.

As Swami Veda Bharati spoke so eloquently that day in sangha at Rancho La Puerta, we are all like drops of water in this vast ocean of consciousness, with no lines or borders between us. Every life does matter, and we are no longer here just to survive but to thrive. We chose to be here to witness this shift of the ages and to inspire and uplift those around us.

We are meant to see each other's goodness and sprinkle joy wherever we go. At this pivotal time, we are meant to use our talents to raise our vibration. As we become beacons of light, others will start to remember who they are and why they are here. We aren't meant to fall into despair. We are meant to rise above with optimism and hope for a brilliant future. We must slice away the fear, despair, and old negative energies and feed our light. Then the world begins to sparkle—one light at a time. With this we will see more and more new ways of connection, caring, and cooperation all over the planet.

Pay attention to your dreams since they can also be a huge support in your journey to know yourself more fully. I wish you so much love, light, and joy on your journey to *you*, your true self.

Acknowledgments

I would like to express my deepest appreciation and heartfelt thanks to so many people who have contributed their time, love, energy, and support for bringing this book into reality.

I am deeply grateful to Arlene Matthews, my brilliant editor, who helped organize my words and masterfully guided me through the challenging process of writing this book. To Karen Bomm, my publishing strategist, whose amazing brilliance brought me through this tedious process of marketing, publishing, and getting the book out there. To Jeff Braucher, my copy editor, for his attention to detail and understanding of the spiritual realms. To Diane Rigoli for her beautiful design work and creative book design ideas. To Janise Witt for her beautiful photography.

My deepest gratitude and love to Phyllis Pilgrim, who was the Fitness director and the Healing the Spirit program director at Rancho La Puerta for many years. Thank you for hiring and trusting that young girl, more than thirty years ago, who was eager for a life change. You helped to change the course of my whole life. Thank you for writing the inspiring foreword.

To Rancho La Puerta, Deborah Szekely, and the Ranch family for allowing me to come back year after year to instruct in Pilates and now Sound Healing. Rancho La Puerta has been my spiritual haven, and it has been a blessing to share my spiritual practices of Sound Healing to hundreds of guests over the years.

My deepest gratitude to Michele Hébert and Dr. Mehrad Nazari, who led me in my initial meditation and yoga practice that continues today. I am so grateful that you introduced me to Walt, Magana, and Baron Baptiste, who forever changed my life. The training continued on with Swami Veda Bharati and his lineage in the Himalayan tradition. You both have been instrumental on my spiritual journey.

To Marcia and Tony Frescura for introducing me to Kundalini yoga, which has been significant in bringing healing to my life, and for trusting me with the crystal bowls in that very first class I subbed for you.

To Mally Paquette for the Kundalini training, human design, Enneagram, ceremony, and astrology, for your awesome understanding of the chakras, and for your love and support.

To all my other teachers on the Earth plane, including Swami Veda Bharati, Dr. Norm Shealy, the Baptiste family, Barbara Martin, Tom and Trisha Kelly, Flossie Park, Sukhdev Jackson, and to the leaders in the world of Sound Healing. Deepest gratitude to Jonathan Goldman, Ashana, Wah, Lupito, Dr. Dream, Mike Cohen, Lea and Phillipe Garnier, John Beaulieu, Richard Rudis, Diáne Mandle, and Amanda Dominitz.

To the late Dr. Mitchell Gaynor, medical oncologist, who has been my hero and support in the invisible realm and who had the courage to share the singing bowls, meditation, and visualization, and to lead clients to sing their soul songs. His work has been a guiding force in my life. You will forever be remembered.

Deepest gratitude to Dr. Pam Laidlaw for our time together and for your voice of compassion, love, and support.

Many thanks to the following people who were kind enough to read my manuscript: my mom, brother David, Wah, Michele Hébert, Dr. Mehrad Nazari, Dr. Beth Dupree, Dr. Pam Laidlaw, Phyllis Pilgrim, Sukhdev Jackson, Deborah Szekely, Lupito, Mary Ellen Capps, Amanda Dominitz, Marcia Frescura, Stephanie Schneider, PhD, Flossie Park, Lea Garnier, Deb Schindele, Jill Nusinow, Barry Shingle, and empowerHER, a nonprofit.

To all my beloved soul sisters on this journey, who have been angels by my side in my healing process: Jodi Fleishman,

Sharon Ricca, Stephanie Schneider, Sunnie Cole, Lily Selph, Laura Gideon, Joy Hammond, Mally Paquette, Susan Randazzo, Dr. Joanie Watkins, Grace Pratt, Carol Swig, Diana Acton, and the Baltimore girls—Amy Suben, Diane Yoffe, and Carol Swan.

To my father, Mitchell, who loved me unconditionally and taught me kindness, smiling, and always welcoming people with an open heart, and who still guides me from the unseen realms. My mothers were my greatest teachers. To my birth mother, Etta, you brought me grace, dance, arts, and named me for LOVE, which guides me always. To Janet, my gifted mom, you put up with so much. Thank you for your perseverance in taking on three traumatized kids and keeping our family together. To Maggie, I love you for your patience and love, and for never giving up on us. You will always be a part of our family.

To my sister and brothers and their spouses: Marilyn Saks, Steven Penn, David Penn, and Art Penn. We survived. But the best part, besides all of you, are your children—our nieces and nephews!

I give thanks to our children: Mitch, Laura, and Eric. Thank you for being amazing, beautiful, kind human beings. May you bless the world with your talents.

Most of all, and most important, thank you to my husband and best friend, Gary, who has sat with me through this journey, answered my million questions, and encouraged me to never give up!

To any and all of my friends and students, you are my teachers. I love you and thank you for teaching me that we are all in the Aquarian Age together in order to expand and become more of who we were born to be.

Whispers' Resources

SOUND AND VIBRATION BOOKS

The Humming Effect: Sound Healing for Health and Happiness by Jonathan Goldman and Andi Goldman (Healing Arts Press, 2017)

The 7 Secrets of Sound Healing by Jonathan Goldman (Hay House, revised edition, 2017)

Shifting Frequencies: Sounds for Vibratory Activation by Jonathan Goldman (Light Technology, 2010)

Chakra Frequencies: Tantra of Sound by Jonathan Goldman and Andi Goldman (Destiny Books, 2011)

Healing Sounds: The Power of Harmonics by Jonathan Goldman (Healing Arts Press, 2002)

Cymatics: A Study of Wave Phenomena and Vibration by Hans Jenny (Macromedia Publishing, 2001)

The Healing Power of Sound: Recovery from Life-Threatening Illness Using Sound, Voice, and Music by Mitchell L. Gaynor, MD (Shambhala, 2002)

The Tao of Sound: Acoustic Sound Healing for the 21st Century by Fabien Maman (Tama-Do, 2008)

Musique of the Sky: Accessing the Energy Field of the Soul with Sound and Astrology by Fabien Maman and Terres Unsoeld (Tama-Do, 2015)

Healing with Sound, Color and Movement: Nine Evolutionary Healing Techniques by Fabian Maman (Tama-Do, 1997)

The Healing Tones of Crystal Bowls: Heal Yourself with Sound and Colour by Renee Brodie (Aroma Art, Ltd., 1996)

Let Light into Your Heart with Colour and Sound by Renee Brodie (Aroma Art, Ltd., 2001)

The Complete Guide to Sound Healing by David Gibson (2014)

Sound Healing & Values Visualization: Creating a Life of Value by John Beaulieu (Biosonic Enterprises, 2018)

Human Tuning: Sound Healing with Tuning Forks by John Beaulieu (Biosonic Enterprises, 2010)

Travelling the Sacred Sound Current: Keys for Conscious Evolution by Deborah Van Dyke (2001)

Healing: A Vibrational Exchange by Wah! (2014)

BREATH AND YOGA BOOKS

The Practice of Nada Yoga: Meditation on the Inner Sacred Sound by Braird Hersey (Inner Traditions, 2013)

I Am Woman: Creative, Sacred & Invincible by Yogi Bhajan (Kundalini Research Institute, 2009)

The Yoga Sutras of Patanjali, translation and commentary by Sri Swami Satchidananda (Integral Yoga Publications, 2012)

The Yoga of Breath: A Step-by-Step Guide to Pranayama by Richard Rosen (Shambhala, 2002)

WISDOM BOOKS

Human Urge for Peace: What Is Right with the World by Swami Veda Bharati (2013)

Whole Hearted: Applied Spirituality for Everyday Life by Swami Veda Bharati (2015)

Living with the Himalayan Masters by Swami Rama (Himalayan Institute Press, 2007)

The Law of Success: Using the Power of Spirit to Create Health, Prosperity, and Happiness by Paramahansa Yogananda (Self-Realization Fellowship, 1989)

Autobiography of a Yogi by Paramahansa Yogananda (Self-Realization Fellowship, 1998)

The Tenth Door: A Yoga Adventure by Michele Hébert (Raja Yogis Press, 2016)

Enlightened Negotiation: 8 Universal Laws to Connect, Create, and Prosper by Dr. Mehrad Nazari (SelectBooks Inc., 2016)

Change Your Aura, Change Your Life: A Step-by-Step Guide to Unfolding Your Spiritual Power by Barbara Y. Martin & Dimitri Moraitis (TarcherPerigee, 2016)

Karma and Reincarnation: Unlocking Your 800 Lives to Enlightenment by Barbara Y. Martin & Dimitri Moraitis (TarcherPerigee, 2010)

HEALING CHANTING MUSIC

Walking Sky, Dreaming Earth by Aykanna with Sukhdev Jackson (2019)

Light in the Darkness: Meditations for Transformation by Aykanna with Sukhdev Jackson (2016)

Celestial Sleep: Healing Sound for Rest and Relaxation with Crystal Singing Bowls by Ashana and Thomas Barquee (2020)

The Infinite Heart by Ashana (2011)

Wah! Greatest Yoga Music Ever: Classic, Live & Unreleased by Wah! (2011)

Healing: A Vibrational Exchange by Wah! (2014)

CRYSTALS

Kayma England, Founder of Kamali Temple; www.kamalitemple.com

Mystical Bazaar in Sedona; www.mysticalbazaar.com

Crystal Magic in Sedona; www.crystalmagic.com

NON-PROFIT ORGANIZATIONS

empowerHER®; www.empoweringher.org

The Healing Consciousness Foundation; www.hcfbucks.org

Crohn's & Colitis Foundation; www.crohnscolitisfoundation.org

About the Author

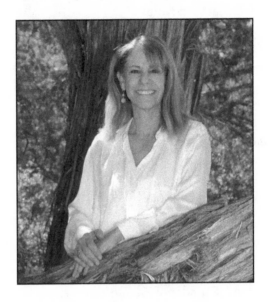

LAURA PENN GALLERSTEIN, was inspired by her "inner voice" to write her first book, *Whispers in Sound.* She is also the creator of *Whispering Wings,* an audio of guided meditations and sound. Laura founded and owns Sedona Sacred Sounds, a facility that offers sacred sound healings with alchemy crystal bowls and guided healing meditations online and in person. Previously she was a co-owner and co-founder of Singing Bowls Temple, and founder of Moving Spirit Retreats. She has been an eclectic teacher of body, mind, and spirit practices for over forty years.

For over thirty-five years, Laura trained with master teachers and leading practitioners from around the world in modalities such as sound healing, Raja yoga, Reiki, reconnection healing, intuition, Pilates. She even has a black belt in karate. She created and developed the first Pilates program at the world-renowned

Golden Door, and Rancho La Puerta health spas. Initially trained as a professional modern dancer, she has taught Raja yoga for over twenty years and currently leads Kundalini yoga classes online and in person. After decades of training and integrating deep wisdom from spiritual teachers and masters with her own experience, she is able to offer spiritual guidance through her courses and workshops. She has a passion for inspiring and educating others, lifting them onto a path of higher consciousness and holistic health through retreats, workshops, and courses consisting of sound healing, yoga, Pilates, meditation, journaling, intuitive readings, and healthy meals. Participants have benefited from connecting to their spiritual nature, improving their self-esteem and lifestyle.

Most recently, in addition to her private workshops, Laura has led sound healing sessions in Hospice and in elementary schools. Her desire is to help everyone raise awareness of the body, mind, and spirit connection throughout the life cycle. Her newsletter, *Sedona Sacred Sounds,* is filled with current news related to humanity's current and ongoing transition into the Aquarian Age. Her ultimate vision is to incorporate sound healing into hospice, hospitals, cancer centers, and wellness centers around the world, and to especially help those who have experienced loss.

Laura lives in Sedona with her husband, Gary and dog, Hop. For more information, visit her website:

www.LauraPennGallerstein.com

www.MeditationsByLaura.com
Access code: **blessings**

Whispers' Offerings

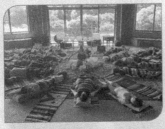
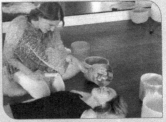
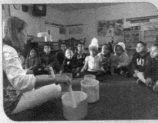
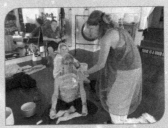

Sacred Sound 3-4 Day Trainings and One Day Workshops

Find Your Voice Workshops

Sound, Yoga and Meditation Retreats

Private Sound Sessions

Sacred Sound Baths

Kundalini Yoga

Sacred Sound Volunteer

Find out more at:

www.**LauraPennGallerstein**.com

Laura will contribute a percentage of her proceeds from the book, workshop, and class profits to empowerHER®

Connect with Laura

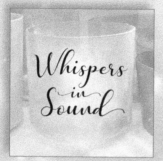
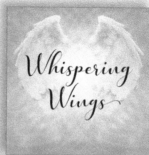

Audio Links
www.**MeditationsByLaura**.com

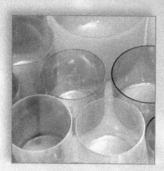
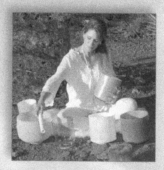

Sedona Sacred Sounds
Purchase your own set of
Alchemy Crystal Singing Bowls

*Receive a complimentary consultation to help you find
the perfect bowl or bowl set for your personal practice.*

Contact Laura: laurapgallerstein@gmail.com

Heal, learn and grow with Laura!

www.**SedonaSacredSounds**.com

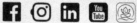

CPSIA information can be obtained
at www.ICGtesting.com
Printed in the USA
LVHW041321110621
689906LV00008B/867

9 781736 559307